For Josie, Eve and Martin, with love (and Betty)

Acknowledgements

The author and publishers wish to express their thanks to the Incorporated Council of Law Reporting for allowing publication of material in which it holds copyright.

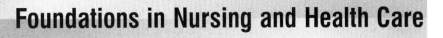

Foundations in Nursing and Health Care

Law and Ethics

This book is to be returned on or before
the last date stamped below

Judith Hendrick
Series Editor: Lynne Wigens

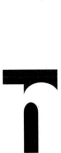

Published in 2004 by:
Nelson Thornes Ltd
Delta Place
27 Bath Road
CHELTENHAM
GL53 7TH
United Kingdom

04 05 06 07 08 / 10 9 8 7 6 5 4 3 2 1

A catalogue record for this book is available from the British Library

ISBN 0 7487 7541 2

Illustrations by Clinton Banbury
Page make-up by Florence Production Ltd

Printed in Great Britain by Ashford Colour Press

Contents

List of statutes

Internet websites

Acts of Parliament: http://www.hmso.gov.uk/acts.htm. This site provides the full text of Public Acts from the start of 1998.

Useful explanatory notes prepared by the government to explain the implications of recent legislation can be found at: http://www.legislation.hmso.gov.uk/legislation/uk-expa.htm

Statutory Instruments: http://www.hmso.gov.uk/stat.htm. This site provides the full text of statutory instruments from the start of 1987.

List of cases

Key

AC   *Law Reports, Appeal Cases*
All ER   *All England Law Reports*
BMLR   *Butterworths Medico-Legal Reports*
Crim LR   *Criminal Law Review*
EHRR   *European Human Rights Reports*
FLR   *Family Law Reports*
KB   *Law Reports, King's Bench*
Med LR   *Medical Law Reports*
QB   *Law Reports, Queen's Bench Division*
Sol J   *Solicitors Journal*
WLR   *Weekly Law Reports*

A

A, Re [1992] 3 Med LR 303.

A, Re [2000] 1 FLR 1.

A, D and G v. North West Lancashire HA [1999] *Lloyds Law Reports* p. 399.

Airedale NHS Trust v. Bland [1993] AC 789, [1993] All ER 821, [1993] 2 WLR 316.

AK (medical treatment: consent) [2001]1 FLR 129, BMLR 151.

A-G's Reference (No 3 of 1994) [1997] 3 All ER 936, [1997] 3 WLR 421.

B

B, Re (adult: refusal of medical treatment) [2002] 1 FLR 1090.

Bolam v. Friern Hospital Management Committee [1957] 1 WLR 582, [1957] 2 All ER 118.

Bolitho v. City and Hackney Health Authority [1998] AC 232; [1997] 4 All ER 771, [1997] 3 WLR 1151.

C

C, Re (a minor) (wardship: medical treatment) [1989] 2 All 782, [1989] 3 WLR 240, [1989] 1 FLR 252.

C, Re (a minor) (confidential information) [1991] FLR 478.

C, Re (adult: refusal of medical treatment) [1994] 1 All ER 819, [1994] 1 WLR 290.

C, Re (a baby) [1996] 2 FLR 43.

C, Re (a minor) (medical treatment) [1998] 1 FLR 384.

Chester v. Afshar [2003] 3 All ER 52.

Clarke v. MacLennan [1983] 1 All ER 416.

D

D, Re (a minor) (wardship: sterilisation) [1976] 1 All ER 326, [1976] 2 WLR 279.

D v. United Kingdom [1997] 24 EHRR 423.

D, Re [1997] 38 BMLR 1.

D (a minor) [1987] 1 All ER 20.

E

E, Re (a minor) (wardship: medical treatment) [1993] 1 FLR 386.

F

F, Re (in utero) [1988] 2 All ER 193, 2 FLR 307.

F, Re (mental patient; sterilisation) [1990] 2 AC [1989] 2 All ER 545.

G

G, Re (adult incompetent: withdrawal of treatment) [2001]65 BMLR 6.

Gillick v. West Norfolk and Wisbech AHA [1986] AC 112, [1985] 3 All ER 402, [1985] 3 WLR 237.

H

H, Re (adult incompetent) [1997] 38 BLMR 11.

HG, Re (specific issue order: sterilisation) [1993] 16 BLMR 50, [1993] 1 FLR 587.

Hay v. Grampian Health Board [1995] 6 Med LR 128, 25 BMLR 98.

Internet websites

The Courts: http://www.courtservice.gov.uk. Recent judgments, including some from the Court of Appeal, are available here.

House of Lords judgments: http://www.parliament.uk. This site provides the full text of judgments starting from 14 November 1996. You will be using the Parliament site, so you need to select Judicial Work and then Judgments.

European Court of Human Rights' Decisions: http://www.echr.coe.int/Eng?Judgments.htm. The full text of judgments is provided. When the first page comes up you need to select 'Search the case law' and then use the search facility.

Preface

That health-care issues are almost always now newsworthy is to state the obvious. Indeed, it seems that we are so preoccupied with our 'health' that rarely a day goes by without some new problem or dilemma hitting the headlines. Perhaps this is not surprising given that health is a subject in which we all have an interest and on which everyone has views. Yet as the 21st century gets under way it is not only the 'big' dilemmas – such as abortion and the treatment of the terminally ill – that continue to concern us. Rather, we are now just as likely to focus on more 'modern' topics such as 'designer' babies, cloning and developments in human genetics. But the potential ability of new and complex technologies to transform our lives is not the only reason for increased public awareness about health care. For what often now fuels our anxiety is growing awareness that, as the NHS struggles to stretch limited resources – yet tries to remain true to its founding principles – compromises will have to be made. In other words, we will have to find a way to fill the gap between supply and demand in health care.

Against this background it is inevitable that many of the decisions you have to make are likely to be more complex than they once were. As a consequence you will need to think very carefully not only about the ethical principles and values that guide your practice but also about how the law regulates what you do. The fact that ethics and law often complement each other can, of course, make decision-making easier. Thus, as you will see, they share the same vocabulary and concepts and overlap in many ways. But this is not always the case. Sometimes the ethical and legal approach to a particular situation is very different. Indeed the difference between what you think you *ought* to do and what the law says you *must* do may tempt you to seriously question whether the law can effectively (or indeed should) control and regulate some areas of health-care practice. Given the rapid pace of developments in medicine the inability of the law to come up with, if not the 'right' answer, then at least an acceptable one is not surprising. But the law's failure to provide clear answers to the many difficult legal questions that contemporary practice raises is particularly disconcerting at a time when patients and clients may increasingly see the law (and the involvement of the courts) as a solution to their grievances.

Studying ethics may not always provide you with all the clear answers either. But in giving you an insight into the moral theories, principles and rules that should guide your practice it will help give you the tools you will need to make ethical decisions.

This book is divided into three parts. The first part (Chapters 1–4) introduces you to ethics and the legal system, the structure of the NHS, caring in scarcity and how nursing and allied health professions are regulated.

The second part (Chapters 5–8) covers general aspects of professional accountability and liability, notably medical malpractice, consent, confidentiality and research.

The third part (Chapters 9–14) deals with specialist areas and includes chapters on caring during pregnancy and for the unborn, the control of fertility, caring for children and older people, the mentally ill and the dying.

The book has two broad aims. One is to provide an overview of ethics and health-care law and the ideas that have influenced both. The second is to provide a practical guide to how they work in practice, i.e. to ethics and law 'in action'. In the course of the book a wide range of authorities haves been drawn on; they have necessarily been treated rather briefly.

In common with other books in the foundation series you will find the following features throughout the text.

- **Key points** – These alert you to the most important ideas, words or concepts in a particular section. Key points are basically a shorthand way of emphasising the main points you need to remember. Certain key words will be identified as 'key words' in the margin in a way that should also help you remember them more easily.

- **Reflective activities** – As you read you will find it almost impossible not to think about your own experiences. The sections called 'reflective activity' aim to build on this process. As a result you should be able to understand more clearly why you acted in a particular way and perhaps even change the way you do things in future. 'Reflective activities' normally (but not always) follow a case study.

- **Case studies** – At the end of almost every chapter there will be a case study. Typically a case study will repeat some issue that has already been covered in the chapter (albeit from a different perspective). But in some chapters an altogether new topic will be introduced. Either way a case study asks you to consider the ethical and legal implications raised by the dilemma (and to compare the two). The intention behind the case studies is to explain what really happens (or should happen) in specific individual cases. In other words they are the most obvious examples of ethics and law 'in action'.

- **Over to you** –These generally encourage you to read other books or articles (usually the original text from which an extract or idea has been taken) that are particularly relevant to the topic that has just been discussed. Because of the size of this book the 'over to you' is useful way of reminding you that it is impossible to do justice to the wide range of issues that a topic might raise.

- **Top tips** – These are added in various places to give you further guidance and help when, for example, a particularly complex aspect has just been explained. Or a top tip may give you further information about an issue (or tell you where or how you can find out more).

- **The relationship between law and ethics table** – This feature lists the ways in which law and ethics, as discussed in the chapter, is similar or different and helps you to see where the two overlap and are separate in relation to clinical decision-making.

Finally I would like to thank Peter Edge, Helen Broadfield, Lisa Fraley, Sukie Hunter and Carol Franklin for their help and encouragement. Their support (at various stages and in different ways) has been invaluable.

The law is stated as at March 2004 and applies to England and Wales.

Judith Hendrick
June 2004

1

Law and ethics

Learning outcomes

By the end of this chapter you should be able to:

- Understand the key ethical and legal concepts and principles that underpin health-care policy and practice
- Understand the role of law in developing health-care policy and practice
- Understand how ethical dilemmas occur and the basis on which ethical decisions can be made
- Critically evaluate the relationship between law and ethics, in particular their interaction in resolving dilemmas that arise in practice.

Introduction

Nowadays it seems health-care issues are almost always newsworthy. Certainly in the last few years rarely has a day gone by without a dilemma exploding into the public consciousness causing either public outrage or concern or even both. New and complex technologies, miracle drugs, increased public awareness and expectations can all be offered as explanations for this interest in our health, the treatment of disease, injury and mental disorder. Not surprisingly, it is the 'big dilemmas' in health care, i.e. issues of life and death, that attract most attention. Traditionally these have been abortion and the treatment of the terminally ill. But now it is increasingly the case that issues such as 'designer babies', cloning and developments in human genetics make the headlines. Extensive media coverage has also prompted public interest in various 'scandals'. The death of 29 babies at Bristol Royal Infirmary following heart surgery, which ultimately led to a cardiac surgeon and the chief executive being found guilty of serious professional misconduct in 2001, is one example. Another inquiry in the same year was at Alder Hey Hospital in Liverpool where a large numbers of organs of dead children had been removed and retained for several years without their parents' knowledge. The inquiry into the murders committed by Harold Shipman – convicted of murdering 15 patients but suspected of killing many more – was perhaps the most notorious of recent times.

There can be little doubt about the ethical issues raised by these kinds of situation. Professional competence was clearly at the heart of the Bristol scandal. Consent was the central concern at Alder Hey. But on a much smaller scale all health professionals make daily routine decisions that have ethical implications. We will look at how these can be identified later on in this chapter. Why the study of ethics is important for health professionals and what we mean by 'ethics' will also be examined, not least because underlying all heath-care actions and decisions, however 'big' or 'small', is a set of value choices that must be made by patients and their agents (Veatch 1997).

The role of law too cannot be ignored. Obviously, health professionals have to adhere to the laws of the country in which they are practising. Similarly, they are legally accountable for their actions (NMC 2002). Knowing where the law comes from, and how it develops, changes and shapes practice, is therefore vital.

What is ethics?

A basic answer to this question is the following: ethics is something that we do every day. It is not only about long words and **dilemmas** but is about people: people with different views, values and experiences. It is about how you can know what you believe is valuable, and stand by that value, and respect other people's values. It is about understanding how your feelings and society's norms relate to each other (Tschudin and Marks-Maran 2000).

This simple definition is a good starting point because is emphasises the importance of values. This raises two fundamental questions: what are values and where do they come from?

What are values?

Values are ideals, beliefs, customs and characteristics that an individual, or a particular group or society, consider valuable and worthwhile. Values are part of who you are and what makes you unique. They influence your behaviour and help you make choices and decisions. They also provide you with a frame of reference so that you can understand and evaluate new experiences and relationships.

Values are important not just when you deal with mundane, ordinary situations but also when you are faced with a moral problem that will require much more thought. So when a friend asks you to lend her £10 to buy some make-up you probably will not need to spend much time deciding how to respond (assuming you have £10 to spare, of course!). On the other hand, if the same friend asks you to lend her £200 so that she can have an abortion you will have to go through a much more complex decision-making process. In fact, you will have to make a **moral judgement**.

As a health professional you make countless decisions every day about how to care for patients – about what care to give, where it should be given, how it should be given and by whom. Some of these decisions will have no moral content. For example, deciding that

Keywords

Dilemma
Occurs when two or more mutually exclusive moral claims clearly apply and both seem to have equal weight, i.e. a difficult problem that seems to have no satisfactory solution

Keywords

Moral judgement
This kind of judgement expresses whether people's actions are right or wrong, and what motives or characteristics we consider good or bad

patients should be bathed before breakfast has been categorised as a matter of taste, efficiency, routine and order (Fry and Johnstone 2002, p. 6). In contrast, decisions that reflect a belief about the value of human life are based on moral considerations and are therefore considered as **moral values**.

So, if you think abortion is wrong because it involves the killing of human life, you may decide not to lend your friend money. And in a hospital setting your views about abortion may present you with another moral dilemma. Suppose, for example, you have a conscientious objection to abortion (conscientious objection allows you to refuse to perform any procedure that is against your principles). What does this mean in practice? Can you refuse to care for a patient undergoing an induced abortion on your ward? You might reasonably object to having anything to do with the administration of a drug used to induce abortion. But what if the patient is vomiting because of the drugs? The dilemma here is that to abandon a patient in distress because of your conscience might impose additional work on another hard-pressed colleague or could possibly mean that the patient receives no care at all. In short, whichever alternative you choose is problematic.

Keywords

Moral values
Constitute a special case of values because they are concerned with ethical issues and dilemmas such as human life, freedom and self-determination, truth telling and confidentiality

Reflective activity

When did you last experience a moral dilemma? Why was it a dilemma? How did you resolve it?

Of course, it's important to remember that the borders of morally significant activity are not quite as simple as has been suggested in the above example. Suppose you smoke cannabis, for example. Is this a morally neutral habit? Some people might claim that it is, while others consider it harmful to health. If so, the decision to smoke can be considered part of your moral makeup.

Having said that decision-making is informed by your value system, it is important to establish how your ideas and beliefs are shaped. In other words, how do we acquire values? Where do they come from? This is the next question.

Where do values come from?

Your particular set of values is likely to have developed over a long period of time, starting at an early age and continuing throughout your life. It is likely that some values will remain consistent while others may change or develop in unexpected ways. Inevitably, one particular value may be more important than another. In other words, there will be a hierarchy of values and you will give some a higher priority.

Your value system will have been influenced by many factors. These include your cultural and ethnic background and educational and environmental experiences, as well as your political views. Your family life and religious upbringing will also have played a major role in shaping your value system. Just as your values will have derived from a wide variety of sources so too they may be acquired in different ways. Values passed on by parents and teachers are likely to have been learned in formal and conscious ways. But some values will have been picked up in more subtle ways. For example, if you admire someone, you may subconsciously adopt them as a role model and so try and copy some of their qualities. Similarly, the values you acquire through your work environment (these can be called professional values) will be those promoted by the codes of ethics and codes of conduct that regulate your profession.

But however you have acquired your values and wherever they come from it is important to remember that the most important step in values formation is one's freedom to choose those values that are most cherished and to give up those that have little meaning.

Key points *Top tips*

- The first step in making ethical decisions is to identify your own value system through self-reflection and introspection
- The second step involves understanding which values are moral and which have no moral content
- The third step is to understand that other people may have value systems that differ from yours
- The fourth step is to identify situations in which some of your values may conflict with someone else's (i.e. patients or colleagues)
- The final step is to recognise that when values conflict you will need to respect the values of others, balancing their values with yours

Reflective activity

Think of two ideals or beliefs that you cherish. Try to work out when and how you became aware of their importance.

Describe a situation in which you felt your values were being challenged. How did this make you feel?

A friend asks you why being aware of your value system is important for your work. How would you reply?

Identifying moral issues

By now you should have some basic idea about what ethics means. You should understand that it is essentially a practical discipline in which your values will help you make moral judgements about a whole range of issues. These can range from mundane everyday situations such as moving patients, deciding who should get priority and so forth, to more complex moral dilemmas such as who gets the critical care bed or when to switch off life support machines. That said, there is one thing you might still be confused about: what is the difference between 'ethics' and 'morals'?

Commonly the two terms are used interchangeably, which suggests that they are almost synonymous, in the sense that an 'ethical' action is one that is morally acceptable. As Tschudin points out (2003, p. 45) both words mean 'custom' (i.e. fundamental ways of conduct that are not only customary but also right). Although we will use the words 'ethics' and 'morals' interchangeably throughout this book you should be aware that ethics and morals can be distinguished. Thus the word 'morals' (and morality) is more appropriately used to describe the standards of behaviour actually held or followed by individuals and groups of people. In contrast, 'ethics' tends to refer to the science or study of morals, a much more academic approach, which has its own name – moral philosophy (Thompson *et al.* 2002, p. 4).

So, how then can moral issues be identified? A simple answer is the following: a matter has ethical importance whenever harm or benefit to persons is at issue. The crucial terms here are, of course, 'harm' and 'benefit'. Other terms and concepts typically used whenever a situation occurs that has an ethical aspect are 'rights', 'duties' and 'obligations'. Often, too, there will be reference to such moral principles as 'rightness' and 'wrongness', 'guilt' and 'shame'. Any of the following types of sentence also indicates that some ethical claim or judgement is being made (Edwards 1996, p. 13). For example:

- That was a good (or bad) thing to do
- You ought to act in the best interests of your patients
- You should have intervened when you saw that man being assaulted
- It is your duty to prolong life whenever possible
- You have an obligation to protect patients.

Having said that these terms imply that an issue is ethically important, you should note that isn't always the case. You might, for example, say to someone, 'You should have turned right at the lights' (Edwards 1996, p. 13). Clearly, both the words 'right' and 'should' in this context are not used in a moral sense.

Other definitions of 'ethics'

There are many ways of defining ethics; some adopt a very theoretical, abstract approach while others are more practical. However, whichever approach is taken – and there are heated debates about the best approach to teaching ethics to health professionals – some overlap is inevitable. That said, the following briefly outlines some of the most common approaches.

Ethical issues approach

The ethical issues approach focuses on ethical issues that arise in practice. These are usually 'big' moral dilemmas that tend to dominate in the media, such as terminating life-sustaining treatment, abortion, 'forced' caesareans, assisted suicide, surrogacy, treatment of the mentally ill and AIDS patients, allocation of scarce resources and so on. Nevertheless, it can include more routine, everyday aspects of practice. Either way the expectation is that legal and policy dimensions will be studied so that practitioners can understand how the law influences practice and responds to technological and other changes in the delivery of health care. It is a very useful approach because of its flexibility. This means it can easily incorporate changes prompted perhaps by a new 'moral panic' about some aspect of health care – depriving patients of essential treatment because it is too costly, for example, It can also easily be adapted for use in a variety of different contexts, to suit practitioners in, for example, community and primary care nursing, midwifery, physical and occupational therapy.

Ethical concepts approach

Typically the ethical concepts approach begins by looking at the development of professional codes of ethics and then attempts to unravel the values that inform practice and how value conflicts are resolved. It also explores various **ethical principles** and concepts.

Some contemporary thinkers (e.g. Beauchamp and Childress 2001, Gillon and Lloyd 1994) believe these principles provide an essential framework for working out moral dilemmas and problems. That is to say, while they do not provide ready-made answers they do offer a 'starting point' for reasoning. The four most widely

⊶ᴛ Keywords

Ethical principle
A basic and obvious moral truth that guides deliberation and action

acknowledged principles accepted as fundamental to ethical practice are as follows.

- **Autonomy**. This refers to an individual's ability to come to his/her own decisions and requires you to respect the choices patients make about their lives (see Chapter 6).
- **Beneficence** and **non-maleficence**. This imposes a duty to do good and avoid or minimise harm to patients. It obliges you to help patients and clients by promoting and safeguarding their welfare (see Chapter 5).
- **Justice**. In simple terms justice requires equal treatment of equal cases. It is concerned with the allocation of health resources and means that there should be no discrimination on the basis of sex, age, race, religion and so forth (see Chapter 3).

Other important principles are **veracity** (i.e. the obligation to tell the truth) and **fidelity** (which imposes obligations implicit in a trusting relationship, such as keeping promises and maintaining confidentiality) (Fry and Veatch 2000).

This conceptual approach to ethics that concentrates on principles emphasises a person's actions and choices. However, it is broad enough to also include what is known as virtue ethics. The central focus of virtue ethics is the character of a person (rather than his/her actions). So, in health-care contexts virtue ethics is concerned with the virtues you need to be a good nurse, midwife, physiotherapist, occupational therapist and so on (Hope *et al.* 2003, p 9). In other words, the kind of person you ought to *be* and not just what you ought to *do* in your particular role. It is an approach that aims to help you know how and when to put ethical principles to work (Fry and Johnstone 2002).

But what do we mean by the term 'virtue'? A virtue is a trait of character that is socially valuable. But a **moral virtue** is more than something that is just socially approved. According to Beauchamp and Childress (2001, pp. 32–38) the cardinal virtues for health professionals are:

- **Discernment**: the ability to make judgements and reach decisions without being unduly influenced by such things as fears and personal attachments
- **Compassion**: the ability to imagine yourself in someone else's place so that you can respond sensitively and with sympathy to their misfortune
- **Trustworthiness**: trust rests on a confident belief that another will act with the right motives and will respect accepted moral values

⊶ Keywords

Moral virtue
A character trait that is morally valued and stems from the motivation to do what is right or good

- **Integrity**: claimed by some as the primary virtue – people with integrity act according to their beliefs and values and do not compromise themselves by acting insincerely or hypocritically
- **Conscientiousness**: you act conscientiously if you are motivated to do what is right. It means not just intending to do the right thing but putting effort into working out what is right.

Before leaving this section it is worth mentioning a strand of virtue ethics called the 'ethics of care'. This approach shares many of the same features as virtue ethics in that it is concerned with certain character traits (i.e. what kind of person you are). Here, though, the emphasis is what a 'caring' person would do in a given situation. It is described as feminist (Gilligan 1982, Noddings 1984) because it claims that women use different strategies in making ethical decisions. These strategies focus on relationships – how they can be nurtured and positively maintained. As such they emphasise virtues such as attentiveness to people's needs; responsibility and responsiveness. What this means in practice is that you ask yourself what each of these caring virtues require you to do, rather than what is the right outcome you are trying to achieve (Hope *et al.* 2003).

Reflective activity

Do you agree with Tschudin (2003, p.1) that 'caring is unique in nursing' because 'nursing is a practical, hands-on-job, where experience, emotion, affection and relationships make up the bulk of everyday work'?

Ethical theories approach

The ethical theories approach is probably the hardest to understand because it is very abstract and theoretical and so seems remote from everyday practice. Put very simply, ethical theories are philosophers' efforts to identify the relevant moral criteria (i.e. ethical principles and **rules**) justifying how people behave. Or, to put it another way, ethical theories do not dictate how we should behave; rather, they offer different criteria of moral relevance and direct our attention to different features of action (LaFollette 1997, p. 8).

Let's suppose, for example, that there are two ethical theories: A and B. According to theory A you must tell the truth. Theory B, on the other hand, accepts that lying can be justified in certain circumstances. So, when you have to make a decision (where you can choose either to tell the truth or lie) you can then justify your

---

⚬━ᴦ Keywords

Rules

Although derived from principles, rules are more specific than principles, i.e. they flesh out principles in a way that makes them more practically useful

decision – for example, to lie to a young patient about the seriousness of their illness – because you have followed the moral criteria proposed in theory B. Remember, however, that just because you have followed the criteria in theory B you are not off the moral hook yet! That's because you may still need to be able to defend your choice of theory B over theory A.

There are, of course, many ethical theories that could be outlined here. To, do so, however, would seriously oversimplify and misrepresent them. The best solution is to draw your attention to the two most influential moral theories in health-care contexts. One is deontology and the other **utilitarianism**.

Utilitarianism

Utilitarianism – which is often famously summed up in the slogan: 'the greatest good for the greatest number' – requires you to take account of the consequences of choosing a particular course of action. It is a theory that is most closely associated with John Stuart Mill (1806–73). If you were a utilitarian you would make a decision, say about telling the truth, by asking yourself this basic question: what would be the consequence of telling the truth? The morally right approach for you would then be to act in the way that led to the desired consequence, namely the greatest good (defined very broadly to include, for instance, happiness or pleasure). Of course, as was said above, just because you take into account the consequences of your actions it does not mean that that is necessarily the morally right theory by which to justify your action. This is because a **deontological** approach might be morally preferable.

Deontology

Like utilitarianism, deontology is committed to promoting 'good' outcomes but, unlike its rival, deontology considers your intentions to be crucial in determining the moral worth of your actions. If you adopt this theory (the most famous philosopher associated with deontology is Immanuel Kant, 1724–1804), you believe that there are fundamental principles and rules that must be followed whatever the consequences. In other words, there are certain sorts of act that are right and wrong in themselves because of the sort of act they are rather than what effect they have or may have. So, the basic question you would ask yourself in deciding whether or not to tell the truth would be: what kinds of duty or obligation do I owe? According to Kant the usual duties are, for example, keeping promises, not lying, not betraying and so forth. This means

Keywords

Utilitarianism
A moral theory that does not regard actions as inherently good or bad – they are valuable only in so far as they maximise benefits or minimise harms

Keywords

Deontology
A moral theory that asserts that, if you wish to act morally, you should never treat others solely as a means but always as an end: it is therefore wrong to treat people as objects

that if you were a deontologist you would be morally obliged to tell the truth.

These very simplified versions of utilitarianism and deontology do not, of course, do justice either to the complexities of both theories or the various different versions of each. Not surprisingly too they have also both been the subject of much debate and criticism.

> 👍 **Over to you**
>
> To find out more about ethical theory and the other approaches to defining ethics, read Appendix 1 in Fry and Johnstone 2002, pp. 162–172. Identify two advantages and disadvantages in each approach.

Why study ethics?

In this final section we look at why you should study ethics. Hopefully you have not decided that it is all far more confusing than you anticipated and so cannot think of any good reason why you should persevere. Remember that this introduction has included some very complex ideas and at this point you should be content if you are simply aware of the main terms, concepts and approaches to ethical decision-making. You are not expected to have all the answers yet. Nonetheless, by introducing you to these 'ethical tools' at this early stage you should become more confident and familiar with how moral theory, principles and values are connected. More importantly, as you progress through the book, you will be able to use them more effectively and so get better at making moral judgements.

Several persuasive reasons can be given for you to study ethics.

- The number (likewise the complexity) of ethical dilemmas you are likely to encounter in health-care settings is inevitably going to be greater than those typically faced by ordinary members of the public in their everyday lives. As Edwards notes (1996, p. 8), in certain jobs you can drift along happily only rarely facing an ethical dilemma – whether to give a homeless person money, for example. But you are likely to face many more in health-care practice. Some will be routine, such as juggling and prioritising care to patients on a busy day. Others, prompted perhaps by advances in medical technology, will be much more complex and may even involve life-or-death decisions. Either way the intuitive techniques we all rely upon when making everyday decisions will fail to provide an adequate moral framework.

- Your patients and clients may be very vulnerable – they may be in pain, anxious, insecure and so on. They may also be in unfamiliar surroundings and so are more likely to be dependent on you for their physical and emotional needs. This means, again, that the usual contexts within which you make moral decisions will be radically different.

- You are likely to come into contact with people from a wide variety of ethnic, cultural and religious backgrounds, some of whose values you may well share. Nevertheless their moral outlook may differ in some respects from yours. You will therefore need to know how to recognise when values conflict and how to deal effectively with such conflict.

Key points **Top tips**

- Appreciate that there are several different approaches to defining ethics
- Remember that however ethics is defined it is essentially about making decisions based upon moral philosophy
- Understand that moral philosophy is the theoretical discussion of what is considered to be good or bad, right or wrong
- Realise that theory and practice function as a two-way process, with each informing the other
- Be aware that ultimately ethical theories, principles and rules are the tools you will need to make ethical decisions

What is law?

It should be fairly easy to answer this question. After all, it is very difficult to think of any aspect of everyday life that is not regulated by some kind of law. The law affects everything we do, setting standards of behaviour even in the most 'private' areas of our lives. But despite the pervasiveness of law no simple definition has ever been agreed by legal writers. That said, a good starting point is to describe law as a set of rules. All rules – whether they are social, ethical or legal – have the same basic characteristics. They are:

- **General**: they apply to everybody, or a specific group
- **Normative**: they prescribe, i.e. tell us how we ought or ought not to behave, rather than how we actually behave
- **Obligatory**: you must comply with the rule if it affects you.

○━ᵣ Keywords

Legal rule

Rules become law when they
are recognised by the majority
of people in a country and are
given government backing to
enforce them, i.e. they are
recognised and applied by
the state

So what distinguishes a **legal rule** from other kinds of rules such as
moral or social rules? First, a legal rule must be reasonably definite,
consistent and understandable; secondly, it must be known in
advance; and thirdly, it must be recognised and enforced by the
courts (McLeod 2002).

An alternative way to describe law is in terms of a legal system,
i.e. a system concerned with 'the administration of justice'. As a
legal system the law is associated with government and so includes
Parliament, the courts, judges, legal personnel (solicitors and
barristers), the police and the bureaucracy that services the system.
Similarly, law is also often described as a process – an approach that
emphasises how the law is made (see below).

But for many legal philosophers the key to the nature of the law
lies in the tasks it performs, i.e. what it actually does. The basic
idea here is that a complex, ordered society cannot exist without a
system of accepted and enforceable legal rules. Law in this sense is
needed to guarantee our basic freedoms and protect fundamental
human rights. One of the mains ways it achieves this is by
providing a framework for resolving conflict. By facilitating social
harmony, law therefore operates as a form of a social contract
whereby members of a particular society agree to work together
so as to regulate their behaviour for 'the common good'. According
to this view, law protects the social values to which everyone
subscribes. In other words the legal system reflects a shared value
system (Atiyah 1995).

There is, however, a very different viewpoint about the legal
system. This asserts that, even in a democratic society, the law is a
form of social control. Put simply, this means that the legal system is
an instrument of repression ensuring that the stronger members of
society (i.e. those with the most wealth) can maintain their power
over the weaker members. According to this viewpoint law operates
as a mechanism by which the property rights and other interests of
the dominant groups in society can be maintained and protected.
In other words the legal system does not reflect social consensus but
conflict (Harris 1997).

Of course, the above alternative standpoints represent somewhat
oversimplified versions of some very different and complicated
political views and positions about the law's role. That said, there is
nevertheless wide agreement that the law can be said to have some
very general functions. These are:

- **To maintain public order**. This function is often expressed in
  the cliché 'law and order'. It is achieved by prohibiting and
  prosecuting antisocial (i.e. 'deviant') behaviour. In other words,
  it makes such behaviour a criminal offence.

- **To facilitate co-operative action**. This is achieved by recognising certain basic interests such as the right to own property and personal freedom. It also provides a framework of rules for regulating activities such as consumer and business transactions. Similarly, law is required to regulate relationships that exist between groups and individuals, for example within the family or in professional and employment settings.
- **To remedy grievances**. In complex societies conflicts are inevitable. This aspect of the law establishes the rules, principles and standards creating rights and duties and remedies to back these up when disputes occur.
- **To constitute and control the principal organs of power**. This process provides the means whereby the authority structure of society is organised, e.g. defining who has the right to exercise political power (Farrar and Dugdale 1990).

Over to you

List of areas of life that you think need to be regulated by law. Compare your list with someone else's.
Think of any aspect of life that is not regulated by the law.
Try to imagine what life would be like if there were no law against stealing.

Divisions within the law

Law can be classified in several different ways. The most common divisions are between public and private law and between criminal and civil law.

Public and private law

Public law includes criminal law and constitutional and administrative rules governing how public bodies such as local authorities, the courts, civil service, the police and other public institutions operate. It thus includes the law relating to the provision of health services and legal rules enabling individuals to challenge how health authorities and NHS trusts exercise their powers and duties. So, for example, if treatment for one of your patients was repeatedly postponed or refused they might decide to take legal action (see Chapter 3). Whereas public law involves the state or governments, private law regulates the legal relationship between individuals (including companies and businesses). It not only creates rights and duties arising from 'private' arrangements such as property and commercial transactions but also regulates health care, in particular professional practice in areas such as consent and negligence.

Civil and criminal law

Although criminal law is the branch of law that attracts most attention it is in practice the least likely to involve you in your everyday dealings with patients. Basically, it includes behaviour that the state considers harmful or disruptive and so hopes to prevent by punishing offenders. There are several different types of crime but all are designed to protect society. In contrast, civil law deals with cases taken by individuals (or organisations) claiming or enforcing a legal right. Typically they will want a remedy – usually money paid as damages. The focus of civil law is therefore compensation rather than punishment. Just as in criminal law, there are many types of civil case. The area you are most likely to be aware of is known as **tort law**.

If a patient was injured because of your negligence, for example, you might face a malpractice action (see Chapter 5). Another area of civil law you might encounter in practice is **contract** law. Employment disputes are contract-based. If, for example, you failed to carry out reasonable instructions from your employer, you might be in breach of contract and so face disciplinary action, possibly even dismissal. Contact law may also be relevant should a victim of a drug-induced injury want to sue the manufacturer or seller of a harmful drug.

In some cases there is an overlap between criminal and civil law. For example, treating a patient without consent is a civil wrong and a crime. That said there are many differences between civil and criminal law, including how the case is started, who starts it, in which court it is heard and what powers are available to the judge.

◕─┒ Keywords

Tort law
'Tort' derives from the French word for 'wrong'. A claim in tort can be made if someone, through a breach of duty, injures you, your property or reputation

◕─┒ Keywords

Contract
A legally binding agreement (which means that you can be sued for breaking it)

> ## Over to you
>
> Think of another example of an action that can be a breach of criminal and civil law (clue: it typically involves how you may get to work and back).
> To find out more about the court system read Hendrick 2000, pp. 7–11.

How the law is made

We get our law from a number of different sources.

Legislation

Legislation is now the main source of law. There are two types of legislation – primary and secondary. Primary legislation consists of Acts of Parliament (also called statutes). Before becoming law, Acts have to pass through several formal and, if they are controversial, fairly lengthy stages in both Houses of Parliament during which many amendments may be made. All statutes start life as Bills. Most Bills are proposed by the government but some, albeit very few, can be introduced by an individual Member of Parliament – one example was the Abortion Act 1967. **Parliament** has the right to pass any law it wishes, although it is now subject to European law (see below). Parliament has this power because it represents the UK through elected MPs (note that there has to be a general election at least once every 5 years). In other words, voting for an MP gives them the right to make laws on our behalf.

Whatever its origins, a Bill can only become law when it receives the Royal Assent. Even then, however, it may not come into force immediately, as it is not uncommon for several months (if not longer) to elapse before it finally becomes law.

Much of the structure, organisation and administrative framework of the health service is governed by legislation, e.g. the National Health Service Act 1977, the Health and Social Care Act 2001. More recent examples – approximately 50–60 statutes are passed each year – include the National Health Service Reform and Health Care Professions Act 2002.

Statutes are known as primary legislation because they set out the basic, broad rules. A more detailed framework is contained in delegated or secondary legislation. Secondary legislation includes several different types but typically consists of Statutory Instruments, usually in the forms of Rules and Regulations. This type of legislation has the same force as primary legislation but is not subject to the same rigorous parliamentary scrutiny. It plays a major role in health service law – in fact the day-to-day working of the health service depends on secondary legislation.

⚷ *Keywords*

Parliament
Can override all other laws; that is what is meant by the phrase 'sovereignty of Parliament'

Top tips

The following steps will help you understand how to read a statute:

- The name of the Act is given at the top (e.g. the Human Rights Act 1998)
- Underneath it will refer to a date and chapter (e.g. 1998, c.42): 'chapter 42' means that the Human Rights Act was the 42nd Act to be passed in 1998
- A short statement about the purpose of the Act follows (to give effect to rights and freedoms under the European Convention)
- Under this is a formal statement showing that the Act has been passed by both Houses of Parliament
- The actual sections of the Act then start, e.g. Human Reproduction Cloning Act 2001:

  1   The Offence
    (1) A person who places in a woman a human embryo which has been created otherwise than by fertilisation is guilty of an offence.
    (2) A person who is guilty of an offence is liable on conviction on indictment to imprisonment for a term not exceeding 10 years or a fine or both.

European law

As a member of the European Union (EU) the UK is subject to European law and treaties. Much of English law is unaffected by membership of the EU, which in legal terms deals mainly with economic activity. EU law does, however, have some impact on practice, mainly in relation to the recognition of professional qualifications, equal pay and equal opportunity issues in employment law. Regulation of the pharmaceutical industry is another area that is largely covered by European law.

An altogether different source of law that originated in Europe is now contained in the Human Rights Act 1998. The Act incorporates the European Convention on Human Rights into English law and as such gives people in the UK a number of basic rights and freedoms that are widely regarded as fundamental in a democratic society. The impact of the Act is that, since October 2000:

- Individuals taking a court case in England or Wales can now rely on the rights given in the Convention as part of their case, i.e. the courts have a duty to take into account decisions by the European Court of Human Rights in Strasbourg
- Public bodies (including the health service) must comply with the Convention.

The rights guaranteed by the Act are mainly concerned with civil and political rights, although several are relevant to health care (and will be discussed in subsequent chapters). These are:

- The right to life (Article 2)
- The right not to be subjected to torture or inhuman treatment (Article 3)
- The right to liberty (Article 5)
- The right to respect for private and family life (Article 8)
- The right to marry and found a family (Article 12).

Common law

Dating back to the 13th century, common law (also known as judge-made law or case law) was once the most important source of law. Although it has long been overtaken by statute law, common law has significantly contributed to the development of health-care law, in particular the law of consent and negligence. One landmark decision, for example, was the Gillick case, *Gillick* v. *West Norfolk and Wisbech AHA* (1986). This set the precedent that 'mature minors' could give consent to medical treatment and advice without their parents' knowledge or permission (see Chapter 12). Another was the Bland case, *Airedale NHS Trust* v. *Bland* (1993), where it was held to be lawful to switch off life support for a young football supporter who was in a persistent vegetative state following the Hillsborough football stadium disaster in 1989 (see Chapter 14).

Common law develops through a system known as **precedent**. Precedent requires courts to interpret similar cases – i.e. cases raising similar legal principles and involving similar facts and circumstances – in a similar manner. What this means is that, in principle, the courts are legally bound to follow earlier decisions. When judges decide a case they make a speech – which can vary in length from a few pages to the size of a short book! In the speech (which is called a judgment), the judges give a brief summary of the facts and explain what the decision is, i.e. the principle of law they are using to justify their decision. In cases where more than one judge hears the case – e.g. the House of Lords where there are usually five judges – there may be five long speeches.

Written reports of case law are essential if the decisions are to be followed and a system of reporting them accurately has developed – called Law Reports. Two of those most widely used are: the All England Law Reports (All ER) and the Weekly Law Reports (WLR). Brief summaries of important cases heard in the higher courts are also reported in some daily newspapers, in particular *The Times* and other broadsheets (such as the *Independent*). Computerised systems and the Internet (e.g. electronic forms of the All ER and WLR) can similarly be used to access up to date information.

⊶ 🔑 *Keywords*

Precedent
The system whereby decisions by judges create laws for later judges to follow; it is based on the idea that it is fair and just that 'like cases are treated in the same way'

The system of binding precedent is based on the hierarchy of the courts. The hierarchical structure of the courts is in fact a distinctive feature of the English legal system and means that, in general, lower courts are bound to follow the decisions of the higher courts, but appeals are usually possible.

Key points **Top tips**

These steps will help you understand a law report:
Re T (a minor) (medical treatment) [1997] 1 WLR 242 (see Appendix A)

1. The top of the report is the name of the series of Law Reports publishing the case (Weekly Law Reports) and the date of the report (1997)

2. At A (see right margin):
   - The date of the report (1997)
   - The court in which it was heard (Court of Appeal)
   - The name of the case (*Re T.*, note that many cases in medical law only use initials to preserve anonymity)
   - The judges hearing the case (three, i.e. Butler-Sloss, Waite and Roch) and the date of the hearing (27 Sept 1996)

3. At B:
   - The headnote (italic); a brief version of the facts and relevant law; this is not the judgment but is a very useful way of establishing the key points

4. At C, D and E:
   - Summary of the facts

5. At F, G and H
   - What the court decided

How the law changes

In the past the law changed fairly slowly. But the pace of change is now so hectic that it can present serious problems even to lawyers, who obviously need to keep up to date. Because of the speed of change it is important to ask why change happens. Take the structure and organisation of the health service, for example. It has been so radically reformed by various statutes in recent years that little remains of the original Act that established the NHS in 1946 (see Chapter 2).

There are several major influences behind changes in the law.

- **Government policy**. Because law is such an effective tool of social change it is not surprising that a new government with a different political ideology will introduce new laws and reform others (sometimes very radically). Typically it will be within areas such as taxation and social welfare that the major changes will occur (likewise education and the heath service).

- **Changes in society's value system**. As attitudes, moral and social beliefs in society change, the law usually responds, albeit sometimes rather slowly. The most dramatic changes in the last few decades have been in our attitudes to marriage, cohabitation and sexual behaviour. Other changes – e.g. legislation prohibiting sex and race discrimination – have also occurred that have been important in shaping our attitudes. More subtle but equally significant in terms of its impact on the law has been the shift in our ideas of responsibility, both legal and moral. As a society we are now quick to ascribe responsibility to somebody when something goes wrong. Whether it is the state, an individual or an institution that is increasingly willing to accept responsibility or simply the expectation that compensation will be forthcoming, our 'blame culture' is now a widely accepted feature of everyday life.

- **Technological progress**. New inventions require new laws. In our technologically driven society the law needs to change swiftly to keep pace. The fact that it sometimes fails – for example, developments and advances in medicine often prompt the most urgent and controversial legal dilemmas – nevertheless highlights how important the law is as an instrument of change (Atiyah 1995).

- **Membership of the European Union**. Inevitably membership of the EU has required the UK to introduce new laws, especially affecting the workplace, so as to make English law compatible with the EU. The expansion of the EU (from 15 to 25 member states in May 2004) will almost certainly prompt further changes (some have already been introduced, such as new benefit restrictions on migrants from the eight east European nations).

These are only some of the reasons why the law changes (pressure groups and law reform bodies also play a part, as does public outrage and/or a serious emergency). You need to remember, however, that the process of change is a complex one – the law not only responds to changes in ideas and beliefs but also helps to change attitudes too. Change is thus a two-way process.

Why study law?

According to Dimond (1995) there are at least 14 reasons why health professionals should study law. Here are some of the most important:

- To know when expert legal advice is essential and must be brought in
- To have an understanding of legal rights of patients as compared with moral/ethical rights
- To ensure that the correct procedures are laid down
- To understand what action should be taken to prevent or minimise legal action
- To understand the meaning of legal terms and concepts in codes of professional conduct.

The relationship between law and ethics

In this final section we will look at the relationship between law and ethics and the role they play in health care. This will involve comparing them to establish in what ways they overlap and how they differ.

Similarities between law and ethics

- Both are usually normative; i.e. they tell us how we ought to behave
- Both are concerned with what a particular society views as right and wrong; good and bad
- Both are forms of social control, using rules, principles and standards to prescribe behaviour and so determine what kinds of actions are prohibited, permitted or required
- Both share a common vocabulary – i.e. terms such as rights, duties, responsibilities, obligations – and concepts such as fairness, justice and equality
- Both have common roots that can be traced back to custom or practice and also Judaeo-Christian religious traditions
- Both influence the formulation of codes of professional conduct and the circulars and guidelines regulating health-care practice
- Both reflect and respond to changes in society's value system
- Both help us recognise the value placed by society on health and the expectations we have of health professionals
- Both legal and moral philosophers spend a lot of time considering the meaning and function of words and phrases
- Neither law nor ethics are infallible techniques for solving all medico-legal dilemmas; rather they both help clarify issues by analysing crucial concepts.

Differences between law and ethics

- Breach of a moral rule does not necessarily involve a formal or official sanction, but breach of a legal rule will nearly always ultimately result in a sanction of some sort
- The law is enforceable in court; morality does not necessarily attract legal sanctions (unless it also involves a breach of the law)
- Some ethical principles are too vague to be translated into law, or the law may not be an appropriate tool for enforcing a moral idea – English law does not force people to be Good Samaritans
- Moral values are personal to the individual and are not always shared; legal rules affect everybody (or a particular group) without exception
- Ethical standards (e.g. in codes of professional conduct) are designed to encourage optimum standards (i.e. the best you can do); in contrast, the law is concerned with deterring bad conduct and setting minimum standards.

Key points / Top tips

- Ethics tries to describe how we *ought* to behave
- The law tells us how we *must* behave
- Studying ethics cannot provide ready-made solutions to practical problems but will help clarify crucial issues and lead to more consistent judgements
- Studying the law will help you identify the legal aspects of practice, the rights of your patients and your duties as a practitioner

RRRRRapid recap

Check your progress so far by working through each of the following questions.
1. What are values?
2. How can you identify a moral issue?
3. Give one reason why is it important to study ethics.
4. Give one reason why we need law.
5. Distinguish between legislation and case law.

If you have difficulty with more than one of the questions, read through the section again to refresh your understanding before moving on.

References

Atiyah, P.S. (1995) *Law and Modern Society*. Oxford University Press, Oxford.

Beauchamp, T.L. and Childress, J.F. (2001) *Principles of Biomedical Ethics*, 5th edn. Oxford University Press, Oxford.

Dimond, B. (1995) *Legal Aspects of Health Care*. Churchill Livingstone, Edinburgh.

Edwards, S.D. (1996) *Nursing Ethics: A principle-based approach*. Macmillan, Basingstoke.

Farrar, J.H. and Dugdale, A.M. (1990) *Introduction to Legal Method*, 3rd edn. Sweet & Maxwell, London.

Fry, S. and Johnstone, M.J. (2002) *Ethics in Nursing Practice: A guide to ethical decision making*. Blackwell Science, Oxford.

Fry, S. and Veatch, M. (2000) *Case Studies in Nursing Ethics*, 2nd edn. Jones & Bartlett, Sudbury.

Gilligan, C. (1982) *In a Different Voice: Psychological theory and women's development*. Harvard University Press, Cambridge, MA.

Gillon, R. and Lloyd, A. (eds) (1994) *Principles of Health Care Ethics*. John Wiley & Sons, Chichester.

Harris, J.W. (1997) *Legal Philosophies*, 2nd edn. Butterworths, London.

Hendrick, J. (2000) *Law and Ethics in Nursing and Health Care*. Stanley Thornes, Cheltenham.

Hope, T., Savulescu, J. and Hendrick, J. (2003) *Medical Ethics and Law: The core curriculum*. Churchill Livingstone, Edinburgh.

LaFollette, H. (ed.) (1997) *Ethics in Practice: An anthology*. Blackwell, Oxford.

McLeod, I. (2002) *Legal Method*, 4th edn. Macmillan, Basingstoke.

NMC (2002) *Code of Professional Conduct*. Nursing and Midwifery Council, London.

Noddings, N. (1984) *Caring – A feminine approach to ethics and moral education*. University of California Press, Berkeley, CA.

Thompson, I.E., Melia, K.M. and Boyd, K.M. (2002) *Nursing Ethics*, 4th edn. Churchill Livingstone, Edinburgh.

Tschudin V. (2003) *Ethics in Nursing: the caring relationship,* 3rd edn. Butterworth Heinemann, Edinburgh.

Tschudin, V. and Marks-Maran, D. (2000) *Ethics Workbook: A primer for nurses*. Baillière Tindall, London.

Veatch, R.M. (ed.) (1997) *Medical Ethics*, 2nd edn. Jones & Bartlett, Sudbury.

2

Structure and organisation of the National Health Service

Learning outcomes

By the end of this chapter you should be able to:

- Describe the main structures of the NHS
- Consider the legal and ethical implications of the reformed NHS
- Identify the main mechanisms for quality control
- Understand the implications of clinical governance.

Introduction – a brief history of the National Health Service

'Creation' of the National Health Service and founding principles

In popular myth the National Health Service (NHS) was created overnight on 4 July 1948 by a postwar Labour government inspired by the community spirit of the war years and deeply committed to 'socialised medicine', i.e. comprehensive free medical care for the entire population. As a unique and radical experiment in state-provided health care – the first in the Western world – the NHS was indeed the realisation of a socialist dream.

But appealing though this account of the origins of the NHS might be, it is not entirely accurate. Thus, far from representing a massive leap in health-care provision the 'instant creation' of the NHS in 1948 was instead a very important (albeit not inevitable) stage in a long process that had started many years earlier. In fact, state intervention in health care had grown steadily from the mid-19th century so that by the outset of the Second World War the basic medical needs of most of the population were, at least, nominally provided for (Webster 2002, p. 2). But state-funded health care had developed in an uncoordinated and haphazard way with the result that services were patchy and inefficient. Standards also varied widely.

What was new in 1948, however, was that a centralised and unitary system – funded by general taxation and based on a nationalised hospital sector – was established (Holliday 1992). It was through this unified service that Aneurin Bevan (the Labour health secretary), building on the community spirit of the war years, hoped to ensure equality of care throughout the country.

The three fundamental principles of the NHS – which defined the basic goals of the NHS when it was first created – were:

- **Universalism**: the NHS should be a universal service efficiently providing a high standard of health to the whole population
- **Free**: health services should be free at the point of use, i.e. collectively financed through general taxation
- **Fair**: everyone's needs should be assessed on an equitable basis, regardless of their means, age or any other difference (Hutton 2000).

Since it was 'created' in 1948 the NHS has been reformed and reorganised many times. The two most important reforms were those introduced by the Conservative government (in 1990) and New Labour (in 1997). The 1990 reforms were based on a 'market forces' approach to the organisation and delivery of health-care services (the so-called 'internal market) that created the purchaser/provider split. They were based on the belief that the NHS could only be made more accountable and efficient by market-style incentives and competition. Following the general election in 1997 the Labour government set out to radically change the dynamics of the NHS. It replaced the market ideology with a consumer-responsive service that emphasised co-operation, partnership and sharing information between organisations. However, following its failure to radically cut waiting lists and drive up performance, the Labour government soon reconsidered its approach and adopted a more market-orientated strategy. As we shall see below, several key 'big' themes drove these reforms.

The National Health Service – in perpetual crisis

Since it was founded, the NHS has been in perpetual crisis (Webster 2002). Long waiting lists, spiralling costs, badly maintained buildings, low staff morale and poor levels of staffing are still a cause for concern, much as they have been for the last 50 years. Mismanagement, administrative problems, lack of accountability and inadequate complaints procedures have all been blamed at one time or another for the failings of the NHS. Two themes, however, have emerged as the most consistent explanations for the crisis in the NHS. These are:

- Compromise
- Underfunding.

Compromise

There is wide agreement (e.g. Webster 2002, Klein 2001) that from the start the NHS was built on compromise. Fearful that a nationalised health system would undermine its interests, the medical profession was fiercely opposed to a unified system. As a result, the government was forced to grant concessions to doctors that effectively guaranteed them clinical freedom and independence from the state. This meant that doctors could be self-employed and that hospital consultants could practise privately – a 'bargain' that has been described as a constant source of tension ever since (Harrison and Dixon 2000, p. 17).

Underfunding

Although in the short term the NHS prospered, it has been chronically underfunded since its foundation, notwithstanding overwhelming public support for the institution. Indeed, polls have consistently shown that the NHS is Britain's most prized institution. Yet despite the NHS's popularity governments have continually sought to contain costs by redefining what the NHS provides. As a consequence, the principles of comprehensive care and services free at the point of delivery have been gradually eroded to the point where individuals have increasingly been left to fund themselves. Not surprisingly, the overemphasis on cost control has meant that demand for health services has almost always outstripped supply (Hutton 2000, Webster 2002).

Key points ~~Top tips~~

The NHS was found on three principles:
- it should be a tax-funded service
- providing universal health care
- free at the point of use to those in need

○━ᴙ *Keywords*

White Paper
A publication that states government policy on a particular topic; in effect, a statement of intended legislation, which may be the subject of parliamentary debate

○━ᴙ *Keywords*

Health policies
Formal and authoritative decisions focusing on health and intended to direct or influence the actions, behaviour or decisions of others

The 'new' National Health Service

Origins

The Labour Party's proposals for the 'new' NHS were set out in two key documents. The first was the **White Paper** *The New NHS: Modern, dependable* (Department of Health 1997). This White Paper was developed through the second major document, *The NHS Plan* (Department of Health 2000). Together these documents essentially made up New Labour's **health policies** (the so-called 'third way').

Some of the key features of the 'third way' in health care introduced by New Labour (to distinguish it from the old Labour party) are summarised in the box below.

New Labour's *NHS Plan* (2000)

The NHS Plan set out health policy for the next 10 years. It promised:

- More power and information for patients
- More hospitals and beds
- More doctors and nurses
- Much shorter waiting times for hospitals and doctor appointments
- Cleaner wards, better food and facilities in hospitals
- Improving care for older people
- Tougher standards for NHS organisations and better rewards for the best.

Source: *The NHS Explained*. Available on line at: www.nhs.uk

---

Key points   **Top tips**

- You can find a brief history of the NHS on the NHS website at www.nhs.uk
- For a more critical analysis of the origins and history of the NHS, read Levitt *et al.* 1999, ch. 2

Structure and organisation

This section will outline some of the major organisations within the NHS.

As before, the new NHS comprises two major elements – primary care and secondary care.

Primary care

Primary care is the term used for all services that are provided outside hospital by GPs, dentists, pharmacists and opticians. It also includes services provided by, for example, occupational therapists, district nurses, health visitors, physiotherapists and so on. NHS Walk-in Centres and the phone line NHS Direct are also now part of primary care. Primary care is the first point of contact for health care. It aims to bring services as close as possible to where people live.

Key points   **Top tips**

- To find out more about NHS Walk-in Centres, visit www.nhs.uk/england/noAppointmentNeeded/walkincentres
- To find out more about NHS Direct, visit www.nhsdirect.nhs.uk

Primary Care Trusts

Primary Care Trusts (PCTs) are local health organisations responsible for:

- Deciding exactly what health services the local population needs
- Improving the health of the community
- Ensuring that local NHS organisations work with local authorities to make sure the community's needs are met.

Primary care trusts are now at the centre of the NHS (controlling about 75% of the NHS budget). The assumption is that, because they are local organisations, they are in the best position to understand the needs of their community. In other words, because decision-making is made at the local level, health services should be closer (and thus more responsive) to the needs of the public who use them. Although PCTs are free to purchase care from the most appropriate provider – public, private or voluntary – they must make sure there are, for example, enough GPs, mental health services, pharmacies and opticians in their area. NHS Walk-in Centres and NHS Direct are also part of their responsibility. Note that PCTs are also responsible for planning secondary care.

Secondary care

Patients whose needs are too complex to be managed in primary care are referred to more specialist services. These services, which are usually provided by hospitals, are used less often and are therefore provided in fewer locations.

National Health Service Trusts

National Health Service Trusts employ the majority of the NHS workforce – nurses, doctors, pharmacists, midwives, health visitors as well as allied health professionals (physiotherapists, occupational therapists, radiographers, language therapists and so on). They also employ non-medical staff, e.g. receptionists, porters and information technology specialists. NHS Trusts are the main providers of hospital services. They are found in most large towns and cities. Some Trusts act as regional or national centres of expertise for more specialised care, while some are attached to universities and help train health professionals. NHS Trusts can also provide services in the community, e.g. through health centres, clinics or in people's homes.

Other key organisations in the NHS include:

- **Special health authorities** (e.g. the National Blood Authority)
- **Strategic Health Authorities**: these were set up to develop strategies for the NHS and to make sure that local organisations perform well

- **Mental Health Trusts**: these are responsible for ensuring that services such as counselling, psychological therapies, community and family support are provided
- **Ambulance Trusts**: co-ordinating and providing emergency access to health care
- **Care Trusts**: these are the key to 'seamless service' for patients, such as the elderly, who have wide-ranging needs. Designed to ensure that the NHS and local authorities work closely together, Care Trusts may carry out a range of services in both health and social care (including, for example, mental health and primary care services).

Over to you

Find out more about the role of key organisations in the new NHS at www.nhs.uk.
What is the role of the Department of Health?

To gain some idea of the workings of the NHS in a typical week see the box below.

Facts and figures

More than one million people work for the NHS in England (2003 figures put the number of employees at 1 282 900). It is one of the largest employers in the world. It costs more than £69 billion a year to run.

The NHS employs 386 000 nurses; 109 000 doctors and 122 000 scientists and therapists.

In a typical week:

- 1.4 million people will receive help in their home from the NHS
- More than 800 000 will be treated in NHS outpatient clinics
- NHS district nurses will make more than 700 000 visits
- Over 10 000 babies will be delivered by the NHS
- NHS chiropodists will inspect over 150 000 pairs of feet
- NHS ambulances will make over 50 000 emergency journeys
- Pharmacists will dispense approximately 8.5 million items on NHS prescriptions
- NHS surgeons will perform around 1200 hip operations, 3000 heart operations and 1050 kidney operations.

Source: *The NHS Explained*. Available on line at: www.nhs.uk

The 'big themes' in the new NHS

In this section the four 'big themes' that characterise New Labour's health policy will be summarised. These are:

- Modernisation
- Consumerism
- Privatisation
- Quality.

Modernisation

The modernisation theme underpins almost all the reforms introduced in Labour's ambitious 10-year plan (published in 2000). It is reflected not only in the commitment to recruit thousands more nurses, doctors and other health professionals but also in hundreds of millions of pounds of investment in new hospitals, GP surgeries and medical equipment. Alongside these developments are major structural reforms – such as the establishment of PCTs and the creation of new organisations such as the Modernisation Agency.

Summing up Labour's modernisation programme, Webster has argued (2002, p. 236) that one of its fundamental purposes was to give front-line staff more power than ever before – the assumption being that, since they were most in touch with the needs of communities and individual patients, they would be able to provide a more efficient cost-effective service.

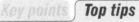

Key points **Top tips**

- To find out more about what the Modernisation Agency does, visit www.nhs.uk/thenhsexplained/HowTheNHSWorks.asp

Consumerism

Consumerism describes the relationship that consumers have with businesses, government, public, private and voluntary organisations. Although it has not developed specifically in relation to health – but is rather part of a much broader consumer movement – it does have significant implications for health care. Thus, as Wallace notes (2002, p. 36), within health care consumerism means a shift of emphasis away from individuals as passive recipients of health care to a more informed, demanding public who expect quality care from health professionals.

As the government itself conceded when it introduced its 10-year plan, many of its reforms were driven by the desire to make the NHS 'more responsive to patients'. In other words 'a service centred around patients, which puts them first, gives them more power and more choice' (Department of Health 2000). Of course, other factors have contributed to the shift towards consumerism. These include the emphasis on openness and transparency, increased media focus on health care, more accessible technology (e.g. NHS Direct Online), greater awareness of individual rights, the growth of health consumer groups and so on.

Although there are positive aspects to consumerism – after all, we all want good-quality, 'user-friendly' services – critics have argued that overemphasising its benefits can divert attention away from more important questions, such as how health-care resources should be distributed in society (Harrison 2001). Furthermore, as Webster asks (2002), do we really want the government to increasingly present itself as something more resembling shopkeepers than rulers, anxiously seeking to discover what their customers want in order to stay in business?

Privatisation

The concept of privatisation in health care is complex and has a number of different meanings (Klein 2001, p. 131). Most commonly, it refers to people (or their insurance policies) paying for services provided by the private sector – such as acute and long-term care (e.g. in nursing and residential care homes). But the word 'privatisation' is also used to describe the purchase of services from the private sector – typically catering, cleaning and laundry services. The most controversial aspects of privatisation are the so-called private finance initiatives (PFIs) and foundation hospitals. Basically, PFI schemes are a way of raising private funds for the NHS. They are extremely complex but seem to offer a cheap way of financing the building of new hospitals and refurbishing decrepit old ones. They are 'cheap' because no public money is needed, at least, not immediately. Foundation hospitals are a sort of halfway house between the public and private sectors.

Private finance initiatives and foundation hospitals are discussed in more detail in the boxes below

How private finance initiative works

Traditionally, when a new hospital has to be built the private sector would build it and the appropriate NHS Trust would pay for it (using the NHS budget). Once it was finished, the private sector would have no further involvement and the NHS Trust would own the hospital. In short, it would have acquired a valuable asset. But under PFI schemes the NHS Trust does not acquire an asset. Instead it buys a service, usually the design, finance and building of the hospital, which is then leased back to the hospital over a long period – typically 20 or 30 years. After the lease ends, ownership of the asset remains with the private sector or is returned to the public sector. In effect, what has happened is that the private sector has given the NHS a long-term loan.

Although cheaper in the short term, it is not yet clear whether PFI schemes offer value for money, i.e. lower cost overall. This is because, just as with a mortgage, paying back the loan can turn out to be very expensive.

Foundation hospitals

The best way to understand how foundation hospitals work is to compare them with an old-style co-op, in which local people, staff, patients and in some cases carers are able to become 'members' of a foundation trust. The members are able to elect governors (who will in turn appoint directors). Within this outline structure the foundation hospitals can establish their own governance arrangements. Foundation status, in theory, allows hospital mangers more autonomy: they are less managed by the Department of Health; they are less inspected and monitored and can borrow money; they can also establish private companies. One of the most controversial features is the fact that they can vary staff pay over and above nationally agreed terms and conditions.

Critics claim that foundation hospitals will create a two-tier system in which the NHS élite get more resources at the expense of failing hospitals. In particular, they fear that foundation hospitals' freedom to pay higher salaries will lead to them 'poaching' staff from other hospitals.

Quality

The fourth 'big theme' of quality has been described as the hallmark of the 'third way' (Klein 2001, p. 207). The idea of quality in health care is not, of course, new – it has been around in one form or another ever since the NHS was first established. But strategies to improve quality had rarely been systematically planned and so were largely ineffective. What was different about New Labour's approach to quality was that it was more prepared than any previous government to confront problems of inexcusable poor performance. Strongly committed to raising standards and promoting efficiency, it is therefore not surprising that the machinery New Labour put in place to achieve quality has been described as its most original and distinctive reform (Webster 2002, p. 247).

Definition of 'quality'

There are many ways to define 'quality'. One of the simplest, albeit very broad, is: 'complying with requirements'. In other words, 'if the requirements of any health-care product or service can be specified, and subsequently delivered, consistently, time after time, then you have a quality service or product' (Emslie 2002, p. vii).

Phrases such as 'quality assurance', 'quality control' and 'quality standards' are also typically used to describe 'quality' in health care. The precise meaning of these phrases depends on the contexts in which they are used. Furthermore, because they are sometimes used interchangeably the distinction between them is easily blurred. When you first come across them you may, therefore, be confused about their precise meaning and effect on your practice. At this stage, however, what you need to grasp about the idea of 'quality' is that it describes a wide range of activities, processes, systems and mechanisms – all of which aim to ensure that best practice is achieved. As such, it involves setting standards, putting standards into practice and monitoring them (Frith 2002, p. 241).

The legal duty of quality

To demonstrate its commitment to raising standards, New Labour – for the first time in the history of the NHS – imposed a legal duty on NHS organisations to promote quality. This new duty (in Section 18 of the Health Act 1999) requires them 'to put and keep in place arrangements for the purpose of improving the quality of health care they provide to individuals'. But the key concept that you need to understand in this context is that of **clinical governance** – a term that basically describes the way in which the legal duty should be carried out (see below for a discussion of clinical governance).

The ethical concept of quality

As an ethical concept, 'quality' is a value judgement. As we saw in Chapter 1, value judgements reflect an individual's personal ideals and beliefs. This means that they are not necessarily universal (i.e. they do not have to be widely accepted) nor are they always objective (i.e. they may be biased). So, although there is little doubt that 'quality' is a something we all want in health care, your definition of the concept may differ from other people's. In other words, there is no one 'right' way of defining or interpreting the term.

◯━┓ Keywords
....

Clinical governance
'A framework through which NHS organisations are accountable for continuously improving the quality of their services and safeguarding high standards of care by creating an environment in which excellence in clinical care will flourish' (Department of Health 1998)

From quality to clinical governance

The link between quality and clinical governance stems from the widespread use of the latter term – in Department of Health publications and in health-care literature generally – as the favoured umbrella term for the government's whole quality strategy (Webster 2002, p. 248). Or, to put it another way, clinical governance has basically now become shorthand for all the processes and activities needed to guarantee 'best practice' (McSherry and Pearce 2002). As such it includes clinical audit, evidence-based practice (see Chapters 3 and 5), clinical risk management, clinical effectiveness, clinical guidelines, professional self-regulation (see Chapter 4) and so on (Wilson 2002).

What does clinical governance involve?

There are several components of clinical governance. Here we focus on two of the most important (Department of Health 1998): setting and monitoring standards.

Setting standards

One of the main aims of the various new bodies and processes that have been set up is to ensure that regardless of where patients live they can get the same health services. In other words the so-called 'postcode lottery' system – where you may, for example, get a particular expensive medicine if you live in one area but not in another – would disappear. Consider in particular the role of the National Institute for Clinical Excellence (NICE) and National Service Frameworks (NSFs):

National Institute for Clinical Excellence

The National Institute for Clinical Excellence has several aims. These include assessing the effectiveness of new drugs, treatments and devices to find out which ones work best and are the most cost-effective. This process may, for example, result in the decision that a new medicine should replace an existing one or that it could reduce the need for complicated surgery. One of the first decisions made by NICE was that the flu vaccine Relenza should not be available on the NHS. Funding it was too expensive as there was not enough evidence that it really benefited those most at risk, i.e. the elderly and asthma sufferers.

Another task for NICE is to produce clinical guidelines (see Chapter 5). Briefly, clinical guidelines (sometimes called protocols) are written plans specifying the procedures to be followed when, for example, treating a particular condition. Rather like a checklist, they therefore provide guidance on the best and most appropriate treatment.

Key points | **Top tips**

- To find out more NICE, visit www.nice.org.uk

National Service Frameworks

National Service Frameworks spell out how services can best be organised for patients with particular conditions and the standards that services will have to meet. They set targets and benchmarks – setting out the care and treatment patients can expect from the NHS in areas such as heart disease, mental health, cancer and diabetes.

Key points | **Top tips**

- To find out more about NSFs, visit www.nsfs.org.uk

Monitoring standards

The main new body responsible for monitoring standards is now the Commission for Healthcare Audit and Inspection (CHAI). Governed by statute (the Health and Social Care (Community Health and Standards) Act 2003), CHAI has several functions that involve both the NHS and the independent health-care sector. They include:

- Assessing the performance of organisations by reference to standards published by the government
- Identifying where, and how well, public resources are used
- Publishing annual ratings of all NHS organisations
- Carrying out independent reviews of complaints.

Key points | **Top tips**

- To find out more about CHAI, visit www.chai.org.uk

Ethical aspects of clinical governance

According to Frith (2002), the various elements of clinical governance can broadly be considered as a move towards a more ethical health-care policy. In Frith's view this is largely due to the new legal duty imposed on NHS organisations to promote quality. She claims that ensuring that someone is legally responsible for performance should result in a better (more ethical) health service, not least because the views of patients and carers will be given more prominence. Furthermore legal responsibility almost inevitably brings with it more accountability. In other words the more practitioners are held accountable – for failing to reach acceptable ethical standards – the 'better' their practice will be (Frith 2002, p. 241).

The problem is, of course (as Frith herself acknowledges), that even if we all agree that improving the quality of care is a worthwhile ethical goal we still need to have some common idea about what we mean by 'quality' (on which see above). Similarly, any process or system that sets and monitors standards – thereby aiming to determine the 'best' treatment or approach to a condition – may be tempted to ignore value judgements or personal opinions about the meaning of 'best', relying instead on scientific criteria – the assumption being that that scientific evidence is reliable (being objective and thus impartial). However, even if it were possible to prove scientifically and objectively what the 'best' treatment is, value judgements would still be needed to help tell us how to use that information (Frith 2002, p. 242).

RRRRRapid recap

Check your progress so far by working through each of the following questions.

1. What are the founding principles of the NHS?
2. Why are primary care trusts referred to as the cornerstone of the NHS?
3. What is the role of the Department of Health?
4. What are the big themes that characterise New Labour's NHS reforms?
5. What does the term 'clinical governance' mean?

If you have difficulty with more than one of the questions, read through the section again to refresh your understanding before moving on.

References

Department of Health (1997) *The New NHS: Modern, dependable* [White Paper]. HMSO, London.

Department of Health (1998) *A First Class Service: Quality in the new NHS*. HMSO, London.

Department of Health (2000) *The NHS Plan: A plan for investment, a plan for reform*. HMSO, London.

Emslie, S. (2002) Foreword. In: McSherry, R., Pearce, P. and Tingle, J. *Clinical Governance: a guide to implementation for health professionals*. Blackwell Science, Oxford.

Frith, L. (2002) Clinical governance: an ethical perspective – quality and judgement. In: Tingle, J. and Cribb, A. (eds) *Nursing Law and Ethics*, 2nd edn. Blackwell Science, Oxford.

Harrison, S. (2001) Right a bit more. *Health Matters* **44**.

Harrison, A. and Dixon, J. (2000) *The NHS Facing the Future*. King's Fund Publishing, London.

Holliday, I. (1992) *The NHS Transformed*. Baseline Books, Manchester.

Hutton, W. (2000) *New Life for Health: The commission on the NHS*. Vintage, London.

Klein, R. (2001) *The New Politics of the NHS*. Pearson Education, Edinburgh.

Levitt, R., Wall, A. and Appelby, J. (1999) *The Reorganised National Health Service*, 6th edn. Nelson Thornes, Cheltenham.

McSherry, R. and Pearce, P. (2002) What is clinical governance? In: McSherry, R., Pearce, P. and Tingle, J. *Clinical Governance: A guide to implementation for health professionals*. Blackwell Science, Oxford.

Wallace, M. (2002) *A–Z Guide to Professional Healthcare*. Churchill Livingstone, Edinburgh.

Webster, C. (2002) *The National Health Service: A political history*, 3rd edn. Oxford University Press, Oxford.

Wilson, J. (2002) Clinical governance: the legal perspective. In: Tingle, J. and Cribb, A. (eds) *Nursing Law and Ethics*, 2nd edn. Blackwell Science, Oxford.

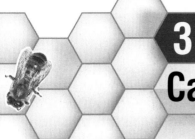

3

Caring in scarcity – justice and access to health resources

Learning outcomes

By the end of this chapter you should be able to:

- Understand what is meant by the phrase 'the fair distribution of health resources'

- Understand that rationing health care is a moral issue

- Describe the various mechanisms for rationing health care

- Debate the different moral perspectives on the problem of scarce health resources

- Assess the role of law in the allocation of resources.

⚷ Keywords

....

Rationing

A process or mechanism for setting priorities in health care, bearing in mind that resources cannot be provided to everyone who demands them; it involves deciding a) *who* should get treatment, b) *what* treatments should be provided and c) *how* should these decisions be made

Introduction

Cancelled operations, growing waiting lists, staffing shortages, too few intensive care beds, expensive drugs no longer available on prescription, once routine tests and investigations suddenly restricted – these (and similar stories) are now standard media fare. Common throughout the 1990s, they are likely to be repeated well into the present century as the UK, along with health-care systems throughout the world, struggles to stretch limited resources. It seems, therefore, that however health care is organised or funded – through taxation (as in the UK) or along market lines (as in the USA) there will always be a gap between supply and demand. In this chapter we look at how decisions about dividing up the health-care cake should be made – how, in other words, we can make sure that scarce health resources are distributed fairly. We also look at the law's role in guaranteeing access to treatment. We begin, however, by defining some of the key terms used in this context.

Defining terms

In this section we define some of the key terms used in the 'rationing' debate.

Rationing

The word '**rationing**' comes from the Latin word *ratio* (meaning 'reason'). Originally, it referred to a process of distributing limited goods and services according to a 'rational' plan so that everyone would receive a fair portion (Veatch and Fry 1987). But more recently the term has become associated with sacrifice and hardship (and wartime emergencies). This explains why it has been replaced – at least in most official documentation – by less threatening phrases such as 'priority setting', 'prioritisation', 'allocation of scarce resources' and 'making choices' (Newdick 1995).

Whatever the term used, there is wide agreement that, while demand for health care is almost limitless, resources are not (Butler 1999). This means that priorities have to be set. Priority setting is relevant throughout the health service. Decisions about how health-care resources in general are to be distributed within the population is often referred to as **macroallocation**.

Priority setting for populations also involves deciding, for example, what sorts of health service should be available. A primary care trust deciding to spend more on renal dialysis than on the prevention of heart disease is therefore making a macroallocation decision. But priorities also have to be set on a much smaller scale, i.e. at local level. This type of priority setting – which typically involves deciding which particular patient should receive a particular treatment – is usually called **microallocation**.

A decision about whether a patient should be prescribed a particular drug is an example of a microallocation decision.

Health-care resources

The term health-care resources can be defined very broadly as anything that can reasonably be expected to have a positive effect on health (Buchanan 1997). As such, it includes medical resources – e.g. medicines, treatments and other procedures such as organ transplants, as well as health education and promotion, disease prevention. It also includes all related resources, e.g. personnel (doctors, nurses, allied health professionals, administrative staff and so on), equipment, research projects and buildings.

Health

There is no universal understanding of the term 'health'. In other words, there are widely differing views about the definition of health and how it should be measured. Traditionally, 'health' has been viewed as the absence of disease but a much broader approach is now generally thought to be more appropriate. Consider, for example, the following popular definition:

> Health is the extent to which an individual or group is able to realise aspirations, to satisfy needs and to change or cope with the environment; health is therefore seen as a resource for everyday life, not the objective of living. Health is a positive concept emphasising social and personal resources as well as physical capacities.

World Health Organization 1986

⚷ Keywords

Macroallocation

Deciding how much of a society's resources should be allocated to health care (which has to compete with, for example, housing, education and defence)

⚷ Keywords

Microallocation

Selecting which patients should obtain care (and for what); it thus includes making decisions about priorities in the workplace

This wide definition emphasises the dynamic, multidimensional nature of health and the fact that it is influenced by a range of factors – social, emotional, physical, environmental and so on (Naidoo and Wills 2001, p. 2). It also develops the idea that health is not a state but a process by which a person reaches their potential (Seedhouse 1986).

Illness

The concept of illness is similarly difficult to define clearly. Essentially, it refers to an individual's experience of ill-health, i.e. what being ill feels like to a particular person. Typically we describe illness in terms of discomfort, pain, distress, immobility and so forth. These 'feelings' can be caused by a combination of factors – both biological (e.g. a virus) and psychological (e.g. behaviours and beliefs). Traditionally, medical knowledge has seen illness as an objective state – which can be discovered and measured scientifically. Now it is more common to describe illness in more subjective terms. In other words, illness is seen as a unique personal experience – albeit one shaped by the values and beliefs held by a particular society. This broader, more self-reflective approach to defining 'illness' is well summed up by Toombes: 'The experience of illness means much more to the person who is ill than simply a collection of physical signs and symptoms . . . rather it represents a distinct way of being in the world' (Fulford *et al.* 2002, p. 393).

Disease

In medicine the diagnosis of disease is largely based on physical findings that can be objectively proved. But this scientific approach ignores the social and cultural dimensions of disease. The concept of disease, therefore, like illness, is value-laden and thus specific to time, place and culture (Caplan 1997, p. 65). To illustrate the way values influence how we define disease you only need to think about the 'horrible disorder' of 'drapetomania'. According to 19th-century US medical texts, this afflicted an astounding number of black men and women. So what was this disorder? An obsessive desire on the part of a slave to run away from his or her owner.

Reflective activity

What does 'being healthy' mean to you?
What words do you use to describe how you feel when you are 'ill'?

- No system of health care has enough resources to provide the best possible treatment for all patients in all situations
- 'Rationing' is often referred to as 'making choices' and 'priority setting'
- The terms 'health', 'illness' and 'disease' are subjective, value-laden concepts (this means that other people may interpret them differently from you)

Forms of rationing – how is health care rationed?

In this section we shall look briefly at the way health care can, in practice, be rationed. Broadly, there are two approaches. First, services can be withdrawn, restricted or denied (as in 1–3 below); secondly, demand can be reduced (as in 4–6 below).

1. **Withdrawal**. In other words, services and treatments previously provided are dropped from the 'menu'. Examples include 'cosmetic' operations (such as varicose veins and tattoo removal).

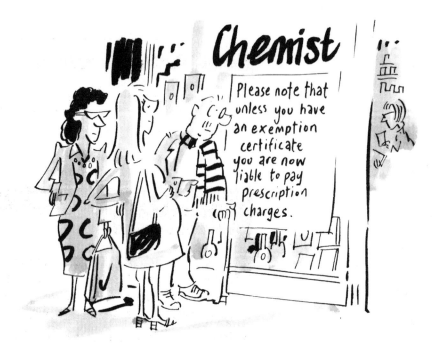

How health care is rationed.

2. **Denial/restriction**. This strategy may involve either denying or restricting access to services because of a patient's behaviour or lifestyle (smoking, drinking, etc.).

3. **Improving efficiency and effectiveness**. This is likely to involve deciding that a certain drug or treatment is too expensive given its possible benefit to patients (see, for example, the role of NICE, Chapter 2).

4. **Deterrence**. Rationing can occur by obstructing the demands for health care by, for example, charging patients (dental/prescription charges); or putting services in inconvenient places so that people will use them less often.

5. **Dilution**. This occurs when no service is actually denied but is instead spread around more thinly so that each patient gets a lesser service. Examples include fewer diagnostic tests or the use of cheaper drugs.

6. **Deflection**. This strategy assumes that most people's first contact with the health service is through their GP. Basically it aims to stop people becoming patients. Techniques used include 'educating' them about the proper use of GPs (i.e. not using them for trivial illnesses). Unhelpful reception staff may also put off potential patients (Hunter 1997, pp. 21–27).

Reflective activity

Consider two examples in your practice where a service previously available has either been withdrawn or restricted. Why did this happen?

Distributing scarce resources – how to make 'moral' decisions

It is clearly important to identify the various different rationing techniques and mechanisms. Yet they tell us little about the moral values and principles that guide decision-making, i.e. what ethical considerations you should bear in mind when deciding:

- How to prioritise your time and skills
- Which patient to care for first
- Which treatments you should give to which particular patients

● Whether you should treat a greater number of patients or fewer patients (with greater need but whose treatment is very expensive).

These are just some of the many examples of decision-making at the coal-face. Of course, you are likely to make such decisions instinctively with little moral agonising. Yet in doing so you are in fact making moral judgements, i.e. judgements that reflect your own personal values and beliefs. Or, to put it another way, you are (albeit subconsciously) thinking about how you can allocate scarce resources as fairly as possible (Butler 1999).

Questions of allocation or rationing involve a range of ethical considerations, including respect for individual autonomy, equality, needs theory and maximising welfare (Hope *et al.* 2003, ch. 13). But underpinning all these is the concept of 'fairness'. So, what does this crucial concept mean? As you will see, we answer this question by focusing on the principle of justice. Justice is the principle that most philosophers accept as, if not the most important principle, then certainly the starting point in the search for an ethical approach to priority setting.

Justice – an introduction

Justice is a moral principle that almost everyone considers desirable – in the sense that we all tend to associate the term with doing what is morally right and fair. But, as with many of the concepts in the rationing debate, it is a value-laden, subjective term (Riddall 1999). This means that how you define justice will very much depend on your own set of beliefs and value system, as well as other personal experiences that help you make choices and decide what is right and wrong.

So, when yet another scare story highlights the effect of limited resources you are likely to ask yourself:

● Why do some patients have to wait longer than others?

● Why should some patients have access to a particular type of care when others do not?

● Why does a child in desperate need only get treatment after a plea by the media?

Your answers to these (and similar kinds of question) will depend on your sense of justice, i.e. how you think that scarce health-care resources should be shared out in society. This aspect of justice is what philosophers call **distributive justice**.

○━ᴨ *Keywords*

Distributive justice
Making sure that individuals receive the care and treatment that is appropriate and proper; i.e. that society shares out its resources in a morally 'right' way

You may, for example, think that a system of sharing out scarce health resources is just and fair only if:

- All patients who need treatment get it
- All patients are treated equally
- Patients are not discriminated against because of their age, sex or race
- Patients get the care and treatment they deserve.

On the other hand, you could decide that it is just and fair:

- To give priority to those patients who have waited the longest
- To treat only those who would most benefit
- To prioritise treatments that cost less
- To prioritise treatments that help the greatest number of people.

Important concepts that emerge from this kind of debate focus on what can be called practical solutions to the many moral dilemmas posed by limited resources such as equality, need, benefit and desert. We will look at these approaches in the next section.

Key points **Top tips**

- You can use ethical theories to decide how to allocate limited resources fairly as well as the more practical approaches used in this chapter
- The two main competing ethical theories that underpin thinking on resource allocation are:
  - Utilitarianism (the greatest good for the greatest number)
  - Deontology (this approach focuses on patient autonomy, i.e. giving patients the treatment they want)
- For more information on the ethical theories approach to resource allocation see Hendrick 2000, pp. 124–127

Justice and equality – the sick should be treated equally

According to Aristotle (384–332BC – one of the most influential philosophers of the Western world), equality is central to the notion of distributive justice. By equality, Aristotle meant that we should treat equals equally (and unequals unequally). In other words, all those who belong to the same group (for a particular purpose) should be treated in the same way. In relation to health care, this means that the sick deserve different treatment from the well, and more resources (Parker and Dickenson 2001, p. 236). But how do we decide who is equally sick? To put it another way, how do we decide which characteristics are relevant in judging individuals as equal?

Of course one way of doing this is to decide which characteristics do not count. Hence most of us would agree that a person's race, gender, height, employment status, income and other similar characteristics should be ignored in deciding who should get medical treatment (Fletcher *et al.* 1995). On the other hand, some characteristics or considerations are likely to be much more morally significant – factors such as medical need, for example.

However, as we shall see below, need is a problematic concept too. How, for example, should two of your patients – who, say, are both suffering from cancer or heart disease – be compared so as to arrive at a conclusion that they are equal (and so are entitled to equal treatment)? And what if two of your patients are competing for your attention and care? If they are both equally sick they should both get treatment. So, how do you select which one to treat first? One possible solution is to choose the most 'needy'.

Justice and need

Providing health care to those who need it seems, at least initially, one of the fairest approaches to allocating scarce health resources. What can be more just than recognising the basic principle that every member of society has the right to health care on the basis of medical need? Furthermore, interpreting justice in terms of need is the approach that corresponds most closely with the founding principles of the NHS (see Chapter 2).

But what does the term 'need' mean? Defined broadly, we can say that a person can be said to need something if without it that person will be harmed (Beauchamp and Childress 2001). Yet if need is defined so broadly it becomes difficult to distinguish it from 'desire' or mere 'want'. Furthermore, just as our perceptions of illness, health and disease are subjective and value-laden, so too are our experiences and understanding of need. It is not surprising, then, that there has been little agreement to date on a set of consistent and objective principles that can be used to assess the basis of need (Newdick 1995, p. 16).

Another difficulty is that that two different models for the determination of need have been identified (Baker 1995):

- **Model 1 – the market conception of need**. This is consumer-led. Accordingly, whatever patients demand and believe they have a legitimate right to claim – be it cosmetic surgery, counselling, infertility treatment – can be construed as an 'unmet need' if it is not satisfied.

- **Model 2 – the professionally led conception of need**. This concept of need is no more precise than the consumer-led one for the simple reason that, as new treatments, services, knowledge and technologies become available, so 'expert' perceptions of need change (and invariably expand).

The task of defining need could perhaps be made easier by simply claiming that limited health resources should be targeted so that everyone's 'basic' (sometimes called decent minimum) health-care needs could be satisfied. But, as Beauchamp and Childress point out (2001), there is little agreement about what should count as 'basic'.

So, although few would deny that life-threatening conditions should be included, where should the line be drawn? In particular, would it inevitably include treatment for conditions – such as infertility – that, while not life-threatening, are nevertheless life-enhancing? And finally, perhaps one of the biggest problems of all with the needs-based approach is what happens when there are too many needy patients chasing the same scarce resource. Who, in other words, should get priority? An alternative (albeit related) approach that might solve this dilemma is to allocate resources according to medical criteria such as the outcome of treatment.

Reflective activity

How would you define 'need' when comparing two of your patients?

Justice and medical criteria

Allocating resources according to medical criteria has traditionally meant assessing the *outcome* of treatment, in particular the probability of medical success. In the past, outcome was typically measured in limited terms – including, for example, mortality and readmission. Now, however, the concept is more broadly defined to include such quality-of-life measures as emotional health, social interaction and so on. Increased emphasis on patient autonomy has also led to the views of patients themselves being sought on what outcomes they expect or hope for. 'Outcome', therefore, is clearly a value-laden and relative term that cannot objectively defined.

Similar problems plague the phrase 'medical success'. How should we define and measure it? As Newdick notes (1995), there is really no objective way of determining the success or effectiveness of treatment given the different perceptions we all have of illness and health.

Relevant also in this context is the cost and efficiency of treatment. This is particularly important when treatment is very expensive and can only help a few patients. In such cases, diverting funds from intensive care units, for example, to cheaper treatments (or even preventive measures) that could potentially benefit far more people may seem a much fairer way of allocating scarce resources.

An approach that attempts to do just this is so-called evidence-based medicine (EBM). The idea behind EBM is that, by using evidence that is of a higher quality, more scientific and more objective, clinical decision-making will become more objective. As a consequence it will be both easier (and fairer) to target resources on the most 'effective' treatments because these are treatments that have been scientifically proved to be the best. Or, to put it another way, using EBM is a fairer way of allocating resources because it relies on science and so is value-free (Wallace 2002).

But is EBM as value-free as its supporters claim? Not according to Frith (2002). In her view, terms such as 'effective' and 'best' incorporate important value judgements in so far as, when we interpret them, we use subjective judgements – about what we think is a good or bad (or better) outcome. She further points out that supporters of EBM also assume (wrongly) that the outcome of treatment can always be accurately predicted.

Justice and desert – responsibility for bringing a condition on yourself

If we accept that EBM is not as objective as it claims, perhaps a fairer way to make rationing decisions is to give people a lower priority for health care if their lifestyle or behaviour has contributed to (or even caused) their ill-health. Giving people the treatment and care they 'deserve' is, on a simple level, attractive since it assumes that people are responsible for their actions and as a consequence it seems only fair to praise or blame them according to how they behave. But as an approach to justice the desert-based criterion is problematic for three main reasons:

- There may be many situations in which it is impossible to assess the impact of a person's behaviour or lifestyle on their health.

- It assumes (wrongly) that we all can agree on what kinds of behaviour should affect a person's entitlement to treatment – so, while smoking, excessive drinking and so on might be included in most of our lists, fewer people would agree about what other kinds of potentially detrimental behaviour to include – e.g. dangerous sports.
- Although we are free to choose different things in life, we may have little effective choice over most of the factors that affect health. Take a smoker, for example – upbringing, peer-group pressure and perhaps genetic factors may all combine to make a person particularly vulnerable.

Examples of patients' behaviour that might contribute to their need for health care

- Lung or heart disease in someone who smokes
- Liver failure in someone who drinks large amounts of alcohol
- A tattoo which a patient now wants removed
- Reversal of sterilisation
- Soft tissue injury from sport
- Accident from engaging in risky behaviour, e.g. hang-gliding or cycling along a busy road
- Accident due to a person's own careless driving
- Heart disease in an obese person
- Respiratory infection in someone who has travelled in a crowded train
- Renal disease in someone who has not controlled their diabetes carefully

Hope *et al.* 2003, p. 184

Reflective activity

Which of the factors in the box above do you think should be taken into account in deciding whether a patient should (or should not) be treated?

Justice and maximising welfare (the QALY approach)

The final approach we consider here has been developed by health economists. It is a theory called quality-adjusted life years (QALYs). Often described as scientific, it involves a cost–benefit analysis. The QALY approach aims to calculate the most efficient use of resources

– that which will improve the quality of people's lives over the longest period of time.

Very crudely, the QALY principle is that a year of healthy life expectancy scores 1 and a year of unhealthy life is taken as less than 1, its value diminishing as quality of life decreases in the unhealthy. The QALY principle compares the cost (in financial and other terms) of different treatments, procedures and health 'problems'. For example, the cost of achieving one QALY for renal dialysis might be equal to 19 hip replacements or 190 preventive advice sessions on smoking.

Questions typically asked in assessing health benefits include:

- How much does a particular treatment cost?
- For how long will it extend a patient's life?
- How does it improve a patient's quality of life?

Note that benefits are defined as improvements in life expectancy adjusted for changes in four key indicators: physical mobility, capacity for self-care, freedom from pain and distress, and social adjustment. Patients who score well on the so-called healthy–death scale are those who are the cheapest to treat and who will achieve the best quality of life over the longest period of time (i.e. the cost per QALY is low). In contrast, patients who are expensive to treat and whose life expectancy is short or whose quality of life is not likely to increase significantly score low marks on the scale (i.e. the cost per QALY will be high).

Several objections have been made to QALYs. A common one is that they discriminate against older people (because the elderly have a shorter life expectancy). Another is that the use of QALYs does not take into account the personal response of individuals to their illnesses and their views of medical treatment (Hendrick 2000, pp. 129–131).

Reflective activity

Which approach to distributing scarce health resources do you think is the fairest? Justify your answer.

Key points *Top tips*

- The concept of distributive justice is concerned with allocating scarce resources in the fairest way possible
- Key terms in interpreting the principle of justice include 'need', 'equality' and 'desert'

Rationing and the law

This section will look at the role of law in guaranteeing access to health care. It will begin by exploring the idea of a 'right to health care'. This is followed by a brief outline of the main statutes governing the provision of health services. Finally, it will examine how patients can use the law to gain access to treatment.

Access to health services – is there a right to health care?

Central to the debate about access to health care is the notion of a right to health. In examining who should receive care, we ask questions about the basic right to health care. Is health care a right or a privilege? Is society responsible for providing health care for all its citizens and, if so, to what degree? These and similar questions are now regularly debated in the media. But what we focus on in this section is whether English law recognises a right to health care. The following statutes are the most important in this context.

Human Rights Act 1998

The right to life (guaranteed under Article 2) includes a right to health care. While this Article requires the government to take reasonable steps to protect life, it is doubtful whether patients who had been denied specific medical treatments could use it. This is because the obligations under Article 2 must be interpreted in a way that does not impose an impossible burden on health authorities. However, as we shall see below, although the state cannot be expected to fund every treatment, the law expects it to act reasonably in allocating resources. As to other Articles – such as Article 8 (respect for family life) or Article 3 (protection from inhuman treatment) – it is again unlikely that a patient who was denied treatment could rely them on. This is because in interpreting them the courts would inevitably have to balance the interests of the community against those of the individual.

Key points **Top tips**

- A refusal to fund medical treatment because of the patient's advanced age could be a breach of Articles 2 and 14
- A refusal to fund because of gender considerations could be a breach of Article 14
- In some cases patients can obtain treatment in EU member states where they would otherwise face 'undue delay' – *Watts* v. *Bedford PCT and the Department of Health* (2003)

National Health Service Act 1977

The legal framework governing the provision of health services is now the National Health Service Act 1977. The Act imposes several duties on the Secretary of State to provide:

1. (in England and Wales) a 'comprehensive health service' designed to secure improvement in (1) the physical and mental health of the people and (2) the prevention, diagnosis and treatment of illness (see further s. 1), and

2. hospital and community health services (such as hospital accommodation, medical and ambulance services) as well as primary health care (such as GPs, dental and ophthalmic and pharmaceutical services (see further s. 3).

In addition to the various duties under the National Health Service Act 1977 other statutes such as the National Health Service and Community Care Act 1990 cover a wide range of other health related services provided by local authorities (which are known as 'social care').

Using the law to gain access to treatment

The combined effect of the Human Rights Act 1998 and the National Health Service Act 1977 is that comprehensive legal duties are imposed on the government to provide health services. Yet almost all of them are qualified in that they only have to be provided 'to the extent that the Secretary of State considers necessary to meet all reasonable requirements'. As such, those exercising them have considerable discretion in how they implement them. This means that when resources are limited there will always be aggrieved patients – typically those who either fail to get treatment or whose treatment is postponed – who turn to the law. This raises two questions:

- What legal options can they use to enforce their rights to health care?
- How successful are they likely to be?

Legal options

There are two types of legal action patients can use to enforce their 'rights' to health care: judicial review and negligence.

- **Judicial review**. Patients are most likely to use the public law action of judicial review to force a health service body to provide a particular service that has been denied. Alternatively, it can be used to challenge how clinical priorities have been set. Either way the claim is that the NHS has failed to perform its statutory duties and has acted irrationally or illegally, or that there were serious procedural irregularities.

- **Breach of statutory duty/negligence**. Actions for breach of statutory duty or common law negligence are basically claims for compensation. Essentially they allege that a decision about the provision of services has been made negligently.

Whichever strategy is followed, however, the chances of success are remote as the cases in the box below illustrate:

Case law

Hinks (1980)

Four orthopaedic patients complained that they had waited too long for hip-replacement surgery because of a shortage of facilities. The Court of Appeal rejected their claim – that they had not been provided with a comprehensive health service – arguing that Section 3 of the National Health Service Act 1977 did not impose an absolute duty to provide health services irrespective of the government's economic policy. Rather, the minister had a discretion in the allocation of resources with which the court would only interfere if he had acted 'unreasonably' (which in that case he had not).

Walker (1987)

A similar decision was reached in this case, which concerned a premature baby needing heart surgery who had had his operation postponed five times because of shortages in a neonatal intensive care unit. Even though beds did become available, these were repeatedly allocated to more urgent cases. Again, the claim – that the surgery should be carried out – was rejected by the Court of Appeal for much the same reason as in *Hinks*, namely that the court would not substitute its judgment for that of the health authority (unless it had acted unreasonably, which, again, it had not).

Collier (1988)

A 4-year-old boy suffering from a hole in the heart who was said to be 'in desperate need of life-saving surgery' had his operation postponed three times because of a lack of intensive care beds. Yet again the court refused to order the health authority to carry out the operation as it decided that the relevant legal principles were no different from previous cases that sought to challenge the allocation of scarce resources. In other words, even patients facing death could not expect a court to interfere with a health authority's decision (unless it was unreasonable).

See further the cases of *Seale* (1994), *Fisher* (1997), *A., D. & G.* (1999), *Coughlan* (2001) and *Pfizer* (1999).

The outcome of these cases strongly illustrates what little scope there is for patients to enforce health-care rights through the use of judicial review (i.e. the public law option). Nor is a private law compensation claim likely to be any more successful unless it can be shown that injuries suffered by a patient were due to a health authority or NHS trust acting carelessly (Montgomery 2003, pp. 74–75). In short, the court's role is not to tell health authorities how to allocate their resources. Rather it is to examine the process of decision-making and to determine whether it is reasonable (Ham and Pickard 1998, p. 74).

Key points   *Top tips*

- The National Health Service Act 1977 imposes comprehensive duties on the Secretary of State for Health to provide a health service
- Almost all the duties are qualified, as provision must meet 'reasonable requirements'
- The 'right' to receive treatment is not a legally enforceable right under English law
- The role of the courts is limited to examining the process of decision-making and to determine whether it is reasonable

Case study

Jaymee's life saving treatment

Jaymee is 10 years old. Suffering from cancer since the age of 5, she has had a bone-marrow transplant, two courses of chemotherapy and whole-body irradiation. Sadly, despite a brief remission she has relapsed. Doctors have estimated her life expectancy as between 6 and 8 weeks. But her father has obtained a second opinion from the USA. This suggests that, with further treatment, there is an 18% chance of a full recovery. Doctors in the UK think this optimistic and consider that the chance of success is no higher than 10%.

Reflective activity

1. Does Jaymee have a moral right to treatment? Consider the following:
   - Whether she 'needs' treatment
   - The chances of the treatment succeeding
   - The cost of further treatment (£75 000)
   - The risks associated with further treatment, in particular the distress Jaymee would suffer
   - Whether she 'deserves' treatment
   - Whether her autonomy (i.e. her wishes and those of her father) should be respected
   - Whether the focus of the decision should shift from Jaymee to the needs of a much larger group of patients or potential patients (i.e. whether welfare should be maximised)
2. Could Jaymee enforce her 'right' to treatment through the courts?

Case study continued

As far as the results of legal action are concerned, this case is based on *R. v. Cambridge Health Authority, ex p. B.* (1995), in which the Court of Appeal refused to overturn the health authority's decision (that treatment should be denied). It did so on two grounds:.

- That treatment was not in the child's best interests
- That the cost of treatment was too high given its chance of success, i.e. it was an ineffective use of limited resources. The court therefore in effect confirmed that efficacy of treatment was a proper legal consideration.

The child did eventually get treatment (paid for by a private benefactor) but died just over a year after the case was heard.

Reflective activity

Discuss whether you think health care is a right that the courts should enforce.
    Should all people have access to the same health care regardless of their ability to pay?
    Do you think Jaymee should have been treated (whatever the cost) because of her age – i.e. should children get priority?

Top tips

- When reading case law, remember to distinguish between actions based on public law (judicial review) and those based on private law

The box below compares the legal and ethical approach to the allocation of health-care resources.

Comparison between law and ethics

- Justice is a fundamental principle both in law and in ethics. This is because achieving justice can be said to be the ultimate goal of the law. Similariy, justice is a core principle in ensuring that limited health-care resources are distributed ethically.
- The concept of equality is not only a founding principle of the NHS but is also enshrined in the NHS Act 1977 in so far as it is intended to provide a comprehensive health service irrespective of age, sex, occupation and so on.
- The concept of need is a common principle guaranteeing that priority setting takes place within a legal and moral framework.

⏴⏴⏴⏴⏴⏴**Rapid recap**

Check your progress so far by working through each of the following questions.

1. What does 'rationing' mean?
2. What is distributive justice?
3. Define the QALY approach to the allocation of resources.
4. What legal options can patients use if they are denied treatment?
5. What obligations are imposed on the Secretary of State under the National Health Service Act 1977?

If you have difficulty with more than one of the questions, read through the section again to refresh your understanding before moving on.

References

Baker, R. (1995) Rationing, rhetoric, and rationality. In: Humber, J.M. and Almeder, R. (eds) *Allocating Health Care Resources*. Humana Press, Totowa, NJ.

Beauchamp, T.L. and Childress, J.F. (2001) *Principles of Biomedical Ethics*, 5th edn. Oxford University Press, Oxford.

Buchanan, A. (1997) Health care delivery and resource allocation. In: Veatch, R. (ed.) *Medical Ethics*, 2nd edn. Jones & Bartlett, Sudbury.

Butler, J. (1999) *Ethics of Health Care Rationing: Principles and practices*. Cassell, London.

Caplan, A.L. (1997) The concepts of health, illness and disease. In: Veatch, R. (ed.) *Medical Ethics*, 2nd edn. Jones & Bartlett, Sudbury.

Fletcher, N., Holt, J., Brazier, M. and Harris, J. (1995) *Ethics, Law and Nursing*. Manchester University Press, Manchester.

Frith, L. (2002) Clinical governance: an ethical perspective – quality and judgement. In: Tingle, J. and Cribb, A. (eds) *Nursing Law and Ethics*, 2nd edn. Blackwell Science, Oxford.

Fulford, K.W.M., Dickenson, D.L. and Murray, T.H. (2002) *Healthcare Ethics and Human Values: An introductory text*. Blackwells, Oxford.

Ham, C. and Pickard, S. (1998) *Tragic Choices in Health Care: The case of child B*. King's Fund, London.

Hendrick, J. (2000) *Law and Ethics in Nursing and Health Care*. Stanley Thornes, Cheltenham.

Hope, T., Savulescu, J. and Hendrick, J. (2003) *Medical Ethics and Law: The core curriculum*. Churchill Livingstone, Edinburgh.

Hunter, D.J. (1997) *Desperately Seeking Solutions to Rationing in Health Care*. Longman, Harlow.

Montgomery, J. (2003) *Health Care Law*. Oxford University Press, Oxford.

Naidoo, J. and Wills, J. (eds) (2001) *Health Studies – An introduction*. Palgrave, Basingstoke.

Newdick, C. (1995) *Who Should We Treat*? Clarendon Press, Oxford.

Parke, M. and Dickenson, D. (2001) *The Cambridge Medical Ethics Workbook*. Cambridge University Press, Cambridge.

Riddall, J.G. (1999) *Jurisprudence*, 2nd edn. Butterworths, London.

Seedhouse, D.F. (1986) *Health: The foundations for achievement*. John Wiley, Chichester.

Veatch, R.M. and Fry, S. (1987) *Case Studies in Nursing Ethics*. J.B. Lippincott, Philadelphia, PA.

Wallace, M. (2002) *A–Z Guide to Professional Healthcare*. Churchill Livingstone, Edinburgh.

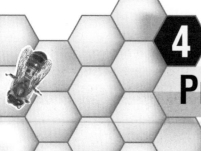

4

Professional regulation

Learning outcomes

By the end of this chapter you should be able to:

- Identify the attributes of a profession
- Understand the legal and ethical implications of codes of professional conduct
- Describe the role of professional regulatory bodies
- Discuss the purpose and impact of disciplinary procedures.

Introduction

Few would disagree with the statement that the relationship between patients and health professionals is based on trust that the latter are competent (Montgomery 2003, p. 133). That this trust has been undermined in recent years – by a series of well-publicised scandals – is also widely accepted. How then can this trust be restored and maintained? As we shall see, this is broadly the task of the various bodies that regulate professional practice – by setting a comprehensive set of rules that members of the professionals have to follow. These rules are collectively called 'professional law'. This chapter will focus on four aspects of professional law:

- The role of regulatory bodies (such as the Nursing and Midwifery Council)
- Registration mechanisms
- Codes of professional conduct
- Disciplinary provisions.

The chapter ends with an outline of the main functions of the Council for the Regulation of Health Care Professionals – a new body that has been set up to regulate the regulators. But the chapter begins with a brief analysis of the concept of a profession.

What is a profession?

Keywords

Profession

A complex, organised occupation preceded by a long period of training and possessing several key characteristics

It is important to explore what we mean by the word **profession**, because there can be little doubt that professionals occupy key positions in society. Indeed, many desirable consequences flow from professional status. These include prestige, power, authority, public recognition and respect. It is clear too that, in providing a specialised service (one that is considered either essential or desired), professions can be said to be meeting the needs of society. A popular way of describing the relationship between professionals and society is to see it as an unwritten contract between the professions and the public. In other words, professionals agree to meet a set of particular needs better than any other group of people. In return, society grants them a monopoly over these particular services. Seen this way, professionals can therefore usually be identified by their specialised training and by their commitment to provide important services to clients or consumers (Beauchamp and Childress 2001, p. 6). But what further common characteristics do professional groups typically have?

Those characteristics that are now widely accepted include (but are not restricted to) the following.

Expertise

Expertise refers to the skills and specialised body of 'expert' knowledge based on research (Burnard and Chapman 2003, p. 2). Expertise is widely recognised as the primary distinguishing difference between professionals and non-professionals. Expertise can be gained in a variety of ways but training will always include

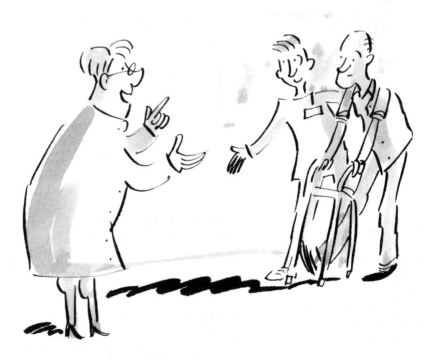

Expertise can be gained by closely supervised practice.

closely supervised practice. However, much of what professionals do also has a strong theoretical basis. Although this theoretical context is not always widely recognised, it lies at the base of many aspects of nursing. Aseptic nursing procedures, for example, are founded on germ theory. Other examples of the importance of theoretical study include psychological theories (which have had a huge impact on, for example, the care of children in hospital) as well as physiological theories (e.g. about giving medication). Sociological theories have similarly had a huge impact on our understanding of the nurse–patient relationship (see further Burnard and Chapman 2003, pp. 2–5).

Following training (both practical and theoretical), the successful practitioner's name will be entered on a register maintained by the ruling body of the profession. To ensure that expertise is maintained (i.e. life-long learning) it is now a common requirement that professionals continually update their knowledge.

Self-regulation

The purpose of self-regulation is to set a country-wide independent standard of training, conduct and competence for each profession. Self-regulation is the mark of collective professional autonomy (Burkhardt and Nathaniel 2002, p. 142). In other words, in so far as a profession is self-regulating it can be described as autonomous.

Self-regulation is supposed to protect the public and guide employees. But, most importantly, self-regulation can be seen as a term of the unwritten contract (between society and the profession) by which the public go to a profession for treatment because the profession has made sure it will provide satisfactory treatment. The 'right' to self-regulation is usually a hard won battle and one that is passionately defended as serving the public good. However, although self-regulation is the norm for most professions it is not sacrosanct. Rather, it is a much cherished privilege – as such the threat of statutory regulation by others (e.g. through watchdogs or direct regulation) is never completely absent (Wallace 2002).

Self-regulation (in its widest sense) means that professionals have the power and authority to control the most important aspects of their work. This generally means they will control the registration process – deciding, for example, who should be admitted or removed from the register and what standards are required for maintaining registration. They will also be responsible for setting (and maintaining) the standards for education leading to registration. Examples of self-regulatory bodies are the Nursing and Midwifery Council and the Health Professions Council.

Accountability

If professions are to be allowed to regulate themselves they are expected to demonstrate high levels of accountability, i.e. they must be answerable for their actions. Or, to put it another way, because the relationship between professionals and the public is based on trust – not just that the latter are competent but that also that they can effectively regulate themselves – individual members of the profession are expected to be both responsible and accountable for their practice. This means that professionals must acknowledge the limits of their professional competence and only undertake practice and accept responsibilities for those activities in which they are competent.

The most common device used by professionals to spell out their responsibilities and explain how they are accountable for their actions is the code of professional conduct (or code of ethics as it is are sometimes called).

Professional culture

Professions almost always tend to develop their own subculture and collective identity. Described as 'a consciousness of kind' the bond that professionals have with each other develops through a common technical language, rites of passage, styles of work and an awareness of being set apart from other groups (Beletz 1990). It also involves being sympathetic, supportive and caring, working closely with others towards shared goals, keeping promises and making mutual concerns a priority. Typically, too, there will be a strong sense of loyalty to colleagues (Burkhardt and Nathaniel 2002, p. 151).

Reflective activity

Consider how long your occupation has been regarded as a profession. Is it important to you that you are seen as a professional? If so, why?

Key points Top tips

- Professionals acquire their expertise through a long period of practical and theoretical training
- A code of ethics is an important indicator of professional status
- Professions are self-regulating
- Professions have a monopoly over the services they provide
- Professionals must obey the rules set by their regulatory bodies (professional law) in addition to the general law that applies to all citizens

Regulatory organisations

In this section we will look at the role and functions of the Nursing and Midwifery Council (NMC) and the Health Professions Council (HPC). Both these regulatory bodies are smaller than their predecessors. They are, however, still expected to take full responsibility for setting and monitoring standards for professional training, performance and conduct. With the health and welfare of patients as their main concern, the councils are also expected to be much more transparent and open than in the past and, most importantly, to take the initiative when accounting to the public for their work. Much has been written about whether the reformed councils (established in 2001) will be more effective and efficient than the regulatory bodies they replaced (Pyne 2002). Most of the reforms have been welcomed (albeit cautiously by those who considered they were not as radical as they might have been). Yet it is likely that, faced with a further wave of public dissatisfaction about the health professions, the Government will find it necessary to revisit the subject of regulation again.

Nursing and Midwifery Council

What is the Nursing and Midwifery Council?

The NMC is an organisation set up by Parliament. It consists of 35 members (24 are elected by the professions, 11 are lay members). Because it is regulated by legislation (the Health Act 1999) it is called a statutory body. The NMC carries out its functions through four statutory committees: the Investigating Committee, the Conduct and Competence Committee, the Health Committee and the Midwifery Committee.

What does the Nursing and Midwifery Council do?

According to the NMC website (www.nmc-uk.org), its key tasks are to:

- Maintain a register listing all nurses, midwives and health visitors
- Set standards and guidelines for nursing, midwifery and health visiting education, practice and conduct
- Provide advice for registrants on professional standards
- Quality-assure nursing and midwifery education
- Set standards and provide guidance for local supervising authorities for midwives
- Consider allegations of misconduct or unfitness to practise due to ill health.

Health Professions Council

What is the Health Professions Council?

The HPC was set up in 2002. The Council consists of 24 members (made up of one representative from each of the professions it regulates and 12 lay members, plus a president). It is a statutory body (governed by the Health Act 1999). The Council regulates the following professions: art therapists, chiropodists, podiatrists, clinical scientists, dietitians, medical laboratory scientific officers, occupational therapists, orthoptists, prosthetists and orthotists, paramedics, physiotherapists, radiographers and speech and language therapists. The Council itself is the prime decision-making body but it is assisted by four statutory committees: the Education and Training Committee, the Investigating Committee, the Conduct and Competence Committee and the Health Committee.

What does the Health Professions Council do?

According to the HPC website (www.hpc-uk.org) the Council's aims are to:

- Maintain and publish a public register of properly qualified members of the profession
- Approve and uphold high standards of education and training, and continue good practice
- Investigate complaints and take appropriate action
- Work in partnership with the public, and a range of other groups including professional bodies
- Promote awareness and understanding of the aims of the Council.

Registration

As a nurse (or other health professional regulated by the NMC or HPC) you are only legally allowed to practise if your name is on the appropriate register. Whoever regulates the registration system is thus able to exercise considerable control over the profession. By granting this power to the NMC and HPC, society is, in effect, conceding a very significant aspect of self-regulation to the professions themselves. This is because it is these bodies that, for example, not only set entry qualifications but also decide when practitioners should no longer be allowed to practise (i.e. when they should be 'removed' from the register). Legislation governing registration is very complex (see, for example, the Nursing and

Midwifery Order 2001). In brief, the legislation covers (among other things) the following key aspects:

- **The register**. The NMC and HPC must prepare and maintain a register of qualified members. They also have to set 'standards of proficiency' and other requirements that have to be satisfied before a person can be admitted – such as the kind of evidence needed to prove that applicants are of 'good health' and 'good character'.

- **Registration**. To be registered, applicants have to have an 'approved qualification' and show that they are capable of 'safe and effective practice'. There are also rules about the renewal of registration, readmission and what happens when registration lapses.

- **Offences**. Details of criminal offences must be specified. These include:
  - Falsely representing yourself to be registered
  - Using a title to which you are not entitled
  - Claiming to be qualified (when you are not).

- **Access to the register**. The public can check whether their health professional is registered by accessing the register.

The new registration system outlined above is far less complex than its predecessor was. In particular, it is now much easier for the public (and employers) to use the register when necessary. More useful and relevant information is also now available than in the past. The changes (and heavier penalties) introduced to the various criminal offences with which professionals can be charged aim to reduce the damage caused by impersonation.

Key points **Top tips**

Important points to remember:

- The professional register is not just a list of names with a few added details
- Being registered gives you the privilege of doing certain things to other people that would otherwise almost certainly be unlawful
- Registration is a public statement that you can be called to account for your actions
- Registration means that you have reached a reasonable standard of competence and trustworthiness
- On registration you will be advised of the professional standards you are expected to reach and what will happen if you fail to reach those standards

Key points *Top tips*

- Control of the registration system gives considerable power and authority to the NMC and HPC
- Registration is an important instrument of public protection
- Being registered gives you legal authority to practise

Codes of professional conduct

As was noted above a **code of conduct** is one of the key characteristics of a profession. Some would go even further, describing codes of conduct as 'campaign documents prepared in a search for privilege and power, or in their justification' (Wilding 1982). Although few would perhaps go so far as to describe codes in this way there can be little doubt that the practice of producing them is undoubtedly strongly linked with the desire of certain occupations to claim professional status. So how can we define codes of conduct? What are their common themes, functions, effects and limitations?

Definition

A simple definition of a code of professional conduct (in health-care contexts) is that it guides professionals in the direction of their duties to patients, colleagues and the wider society (Tschudin 1996). Building on this we can say that codes are **normative**.

As such they describe – with varying degrees of detail – the expectations placed upon and the behaviour required of practitioners within a particular profession. In so doing they state the ideal professional standards and set out the general rights, duties and policies that should govern professional practice. Codes of professional conduct are the principal way that bodies such as the NMC and HPC carry out their statutory duty to provide advice on standards of professional conduct (Montgomery 2003, p. 162). Codes of professional conduct are often referred to as codes of ethics. This is because, in describing the moral standards that should guide your professional conduct, they embody the ethics of a particular profession (i.e. **professional ethics**) rather than your own **personal ethics**.

Functions

Codes of professional conduct usually begin with describing their functions. Despite variations in emphasis, most have broadly the same purposes. These are:

⦿━ Keywords

Code of professional conduct

Lays down broad principles that should underpin practice; as such it provides a framework to guide professional action

⦿━ Keywords

Normative

Concerned with describing what should be done and how you should behave; i.e. the moral principles, rules and values that should guide your actions

⦿━ Keywords

Professional ethics

The agreed standards and behaviours expected of members of a given professional group

⦿━ Keywords

Personal ethics

Your personal morality and set of moral values, i.e. those you choose to live by and which generally guide your behaviour and conscience

- **To set, maintain and improve ethical standards**. One of the main ways codes achieve this is by giving advice and guidance to professionals about their duties and moral responsibilities. Similarly, they advise practitioners of patients' rights and the consequence of unethical behaviour.

- **To regulate ethical professional conduct**. Because codes set standards of ethical practice – telling professionals what kinds of action are permitted, prohibited or required – the boundaries of acceptable and unacceptable moral behaviour are made clear. Practitioners thus know what is expected of them.

- **To provide information**. As a public statement, codes are the main vehicle for informing the public, other professions and employees about the standards that professionals are expected to reach.

- **To encourage a common identity**. Codes help foster and reinforce a professional subculture that binds members together and encourages a strong sense of unity and commitment to shared goals.

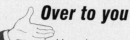

Over to you

How does your code of conduct describe its functions?

Common themes

Several themes recur in all health-care professional codes. These can be broadly grouped into three categories.

Professional issues

These include the following duties and responsibilities:

- To co-operate with others (e.g. patients, their families and other health professionals)
- To maintain professional competence and knowledge
- To behave in a way that upholds the reputation of the profession
- To promote a safe working environment (i.e. responsibility for reporting incompetent colleagues or unsafe practices)
- Personal accountability for practice.

Patient issues

These focus on the following duties:

- To respect patients as individuals

- To uphold patient confidentiality
- To respect patient autonomy (i.e. obtain consent to treatment)
- Not to discriminate (on basis of gender, age, race, religion, etc.)
- To minimise risks to patients.

Societal issues

These emphasise duties to the wider community and typically include:

- An obligation to protect and support the health of the community
- A recognition of the duty to obey the laws of the country in which the heath professional practises.

Effects

Although codes of conduct are not legally binding, i.e. they are not law in the way that a statute is law, they are nevertheless very important documents. This is because they are frequently used as the basis against which allegations of professional misconduct or incompetence are judged. In other words if you breach one (or more) of the rules you may face:

- Disciplinary action by the NMC or HPC (see below)
- Legal action, for example, a negligence claim (see Chapter 5).

Key points | **Top tips**

- Be aware that a wide range of standards and guidance publications can expand upon (and develop) professional issues and themes identified in codes of professional conduct
- A list of current publications is available from your regulatory body's website, e.g. www.nmc-uk.org
- The exception to the general rule that codes of conduct are not legally binding is the Midwives Rules (1998)

Limitations

As Tschudin (2003, p. 71) wisely observes, the ideal code will perhaps never exist; after all, codes have to satisfy a vast number of people and interests. That said, the three major limitations of almost all codes of ethics are:

- **Generality**. In setting out general rights, duties, values and policies, codes may be of little use to anyone hoping to find the answer to a specific moral problem or dilemma. In other words, they may be useful as a broad, albeit vague, guide to the ideal (i.e. best possible) standards expected but little use in providing guidance in a specific situation.

- **Oversimplification**. Codes tend to oversimplify moral values, rules and principles. As a consequence, practitioners may assume that they are more authoritative than they really are. If this happens, there is a very real danger that they can become an unreliable reference point – encouraging professionals to believe (falsely) that they have acted 'morally', i.e. that they have taken the 'right' action (Beauchamp and Childress 2001, p. 6).

- **They are time-specific**. Although codes may seem comprehensive when they are first published, it is important to remember that they are not 'written in stone' (Tschudin 2003, p. 93). In other words, they must be regularly updated and amended to reflect both changes in the professions themselves and changes in society. Thus, although the UKCC (the predecessor to the NMC) code lasted for 10 years it is too soon to tell whether its replacement (the current NMC 2002 version) will last that long.

> ### *Over to you*
>
> Read Tschudin 2003, pp. 88–98 for a detailed discussion of the clauses in the NMC Code of Professional Conduct 2002

Key points Top tips

- Codes of conduct are commonly referred to as codes of ethics
- Codes tell professionals how they *ought* to behave and how they *must* behave
- Codes emphasise the personal accountability of professionals
- Codes do not have the force of statute but their breach can have serious consequences

---

Disciplinary procedures

In this section we outline the disciplinary mechanisms of the NMC (those of the HPC are broadly the same). Bearing in mind that self-regulation claims to protect the public (see above), it is self-evident that, to be seen to be effective, disciplinary procedures must not be driven by professional self-interests. On the other hand, neither should punishment of individual practitioners be their primary aim. Rather, as Pyne has argued (1995, p. 48), disciplinary procedures should:

> be seen in positive terms – as one of the ways in which a regulatory body, acting on behalf of the profession, honours the contract between the profession and society by ensuring that any member of the profession who has failed to meet the trust which society has placed in him or her is not permitted to continue to practise, or, if the failure has been a serious one, [s/he] is reminded of the standard which professional practitioners are expected to meet . . . .

The legislation governing the disciplinary procedures was radically reformed in 2002. Although detailed and complex, in essence the new scheme aims to ensure that action is taken whenever a health professional's fitness to practise is impaired, by reason of misconduct, lack of competence, ill health, criminal conviction or cautions. Explaining what this means, the NMC states that it includes:

- Failing always to put a patient's interests first
- Not being properly trained, qualified and up to date
- Failing to treat patients with respect and dignity
- Not speaking up for patients who cannot speak for themselves.

So what specific kinds of behaviour are likely to prompt disciplinary action?

'Disciplinary' actions

According to the NMC (2002) the most common examples are:

- Physical, sexual or verbal abuse of patients (i.e. hitting, shouting or swearing)
- Stealing money or property from patients
- Failing to care for patients properly (i.e. failing to make sure they are getting proper food or drink or that they are clean)
- Failing to keep proper records
- Giving patients drugs in a dangerous way
- Deliberately concealing unsafe practice
- Committing criminal offences
- Alcohol or drug dependence

- Untreated mental illness
- Serious personality disorder.

Procedure

Once an allegation (or complaint) has been made, certain set procedures must be followed.

The simplest way to explain the disciplinary process is to divide it into two stages. The first is the preliminary (or screening) stage. This basically involves deciding whether the complaint or allegation is well founded. If it is not, the case will be closed and no further action will be taken. If, on the other hand, there is a case to answer, a range of options are available including mediation or referral for a full hearing.

At the second stage, when, for example, a full hearing takes place to decide whether 'misconduct' (i.e. behaviour that is 'unworthy') has occurred, three separate questions have to be considered:

- What exactly happened, i.e. what are the facts of the case?
- Does what happened makes the health professional unfit to practise?
- What action should be taken?

Alternatively, if it is alleged that a health professional is unfit to practise through ill health, e.g. is mentally ill or alcohol- or drug-dependent, different procedures have to be followed. These include the appointment of medical assessors and, when necessary, witnesses.

Sanctions

If the allegation (of misconduct or ill-health) is 'proved', several sanctions are available:

- Mediation
- Decision that no further action is necessary
- A striking-off order, which removes a person's name from the register so that s/he can no longer practise
- A suspension order, which means that a person cannot practise for a specified period (up to a year or less)
- Condition of practice order, which imposes conditions (lasting up to 3 years)
- Caution (lasting up to 5 years).

Note that appeals – to an appropriate court – are possible against any of the above sanctions. It is also possible for a person who has been struck off the register to apply to be restored.

Reflective activity

Would any of the following count as misconduct by your professional body:

- Committing adultery
- Being found guilty of breach of the peace after being involved in a political demonstration
- Shop-lifting
- A conviction for dangerous driving
- Being drunk while off duty?

Key points | Top tips

- Disciplinary procedures cover cases where complaints or allegations are made that health professionals are unfit to practise
- Fitness can be impaired by misconduct, lack of competence, ill health or criminal convictions or cautions
- If found guilty, health professionals can face a range of sanctions, some of which may prevent them from continuing to practise

Regulating the NMC and HPC – the Council for the Regulation of Health Care

Professionals

One of the many recommendations to emerge from the Kennedy Inquiry (2001) into the death of 29 babies at Bristol Royal Infirmary after cardiac surgery was the need for an overarching body for the regulation of health professionals – a body that should be independent from the professions and from government. This led to a new body, the Council for the Regulation of Health Care Professionals (CRHCP), being set up in 2002. The Council does not replace the NMC or HPC, or the other professional bodies that it regulates (doctors, dentists, opticians, osteopaths, chiropractors and pharmacists). Rather, its role is to oversee the work of existing regulatory bodies, thereby building a new framework for self-regulation. In particular, it is expected to make sure that secrecy and lack of accountability – which were at the heart of several of the worst scandals that hit the headlines throughout the 1990s – never recur.

To restore the public's confidence in the ability of professions to regulate themselves effectively, the Council has a variety of powers backed by statutory functions (contained in the National Health Service Reform and Health Care Professions Act 2002).

Broadly (see further Part 2 of the Act), the Council's functions are:

- To put patients' interests first
- To be open and transparent and allow robust public scrutiny
- To be responsive to change
- To provide for greater integration and co-ordination between the regulatory bodies and the sharing of good practice and information
- To require the regulatory bodies to conform to principles of good regulation
- To ensure that the regulatory bodies act in a more consistent manner.

Although generally welcomed by health professionals as a long overdue reform, some commentators (e.g. Montgomery 2003, p. 136) remain unconvinced by the new system. Montgomery suggests, for example, that the system is not radical enough and will fail to put in place a new type of interprofessional regulating body. Furthermore, with so many (possibly conflicting) roles it is more than likely that none will be carried out effectively.

Whether any of these criticisms are valid will, of course, only become evident in time. But there can be little doubt that structures are now in place that have the potential to give government greater control of the health-care professions than was possible in the past (Mason *et al.* 2002, p. 18).

Key points   *Top tips*

- The Council for the Regulation of Health Care Professionals oversees the NMC and HPC (among other regulatory bodies)
- The Council has been created to ensure that those bodies promote the interests of patients and the public

---

ᴿᴿᴿᴿᴿ**Rapid recap**

Check your progress so far by working through each of the following questions.

1. What is professional law?
2. What are the main functions of codes of professional conduct?
3. What do the NMC and HPC do?
4. When is a health professional's 'fitness to practise' impaired?
5. What is the Council for the Regulation of Health Care Professionals?

If you have difficulty with more than one of the questions, read through the section again to refresh your understanding before moving on.

References

Beauchamp, T.L. and Childress, J.F. (2001) *Principles of Biomedical Ethics*, 5th edn. Oxford University Press, Oxford.

Beletz, E. (1990) The evolving profession: the role of the professional organisation. In: *The Nursing Profession: Turning Points* (ed. N.L. Chaska). C.V. Mosby, St Louis, MO.

Burkhardt, M.A. and Nathaniel, A.K. (2002) *Ethics and Issues in Contemporary Nursing*, 2nd edn. Delmar, Albany, NY.

Burnard, P. and Chapman, C. (2003) *Professional and Ethical Issues in Nursing*, 3rd edn. Baillière Tindall, Edinburgh.

Mason, J.K., McCall Smith, R.A. and Laurie, G.T. (2002) *Law and Medical Ethics*, 6th edn. Butterworths, London.

Montgomery, J. (2003) *Health Care Law*. Oxford University Press, Oxford.

Pyne, R. (1995) The professional dimension. In: *Nursing Law and Ethics* (eds J. Tingle and A. Cribb). Blackwell Science, Oxford.

Pyne, R. (2002) The professional dimension: professional regulation in nursing, midwifery and health visiting. In: *Nursing Law and Ethics*, 2nd edn (eds J. Tingle and A. Cribb). Blackwell Science, Oxford.

Tschudin, V. (1996) *Ethics, Nurses and Patients*. Baillière Tindall, London.

Tschudin V. (2003) *Ethics in Nursing: The caring relationship*, 3rd edn, Butterworth Heinemann, Edinburgh.

Wallace, M. (2002) *A–Z Guide to Professional Healthcare*. Churchill Livingstone, Edinburgh.

Wilding, P. (1982) *Professional Power and Social Welfare*. Routledge & Kegan Paul, London.

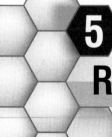

5

Responsibility, accountability and negligence

Learning outcomes

By the end of this chapter you should be able to:

- Understand (and distinguish between) the legal and ethical concepts of accountability and responsibility
- Discuss the principles of beneficence and non-maleficence
- Describe the basic elements of a negligence action
- Explain how the principle of fault underpins the law of negligence.

Introduction

We live in a society where demands for accountability and 'taking responsibility' are so commonplace that pinning the blame on someone or something has become almost a gut reaction. This chapter explores why this culture of blame is so widespread in the NHS – why, in short, there are no longer any accidents or mistakes, as somebody (or something) must be made to answer for 'what went wrong'.

In examining the factors behind the dramatic rise in malpractice claims (and complaints) against health professionals we will discuss the concepts of responsibility and accountability – in both their moral and legal form. We also discuss the law of negligence and current reform proposals. But we begin by outlining two key moral principles: beneficence and non-maleficence. These two principles provide the moral foundations for the various obligations in your code of professional conduct. They also underpin the concept of fault – which, as we shall see, lies at the heart of negligence law.

Beneficence

O━π Keywords

....

Beneficence

'Doing good'; includes actions, attitudes and values of caring such as compassion, competence, conscience, commitment, empathy and sympathy

In health-care situations the principle of beneficence initially seems very straightforward. This is because in a very general sense **beneficence** means that you must act in ways that benefit others. Often summed up simply as the duty to care, beneficence is a stringent requirement that imposes a positive moral obligation on you, i.e. you must help other people. Indeed, as a professional, you have both a moral and legal duty – to 'do good'. But although there is no doubt that beneficence is a major part of your duty as a professional, working out precisely how you are supposed to positively benefit others – i.e. how you must act in practice – is a much more difficult task. In other words, we need to find out what counts as a benefit. Far from clear, too, is to whom you owe positive moral obligations, i.e. who you must benefit.

Defining 'benefit'

There are various ways of defining 'benefit'. Usually, terms such as 'well-being', 'interests' and 'health' are used interchangeably to explain the 'good' that you are expected to promote. Such words cover both physical and psychological benefits, in particular the prevention of illness and disease, the restoration of health and the reduction of pain and suffering (Fry and Johnstone 2002). Yet all these are subjective terms that depend on an each individual's evaluation of the situation and that individual's particular beliefs and values. In other words, what counts as a benefit (or good) and how it is assessed cannot be objectively determined given the different attitudes we can have towards illness, disease, pain, disability and so on (see Chapter 3).

A related question is whether health benefits (likewise 'well-being' and 'interests') should be broadly interpreted to include social, economic, religious and spiritual benefits. If the wide definition of health suggested by the World Health Organization (1986) is accepted (see Chapter 3) then the answer must surely be yes.

Who must you benefit?

There is no doubt that your primary (i.e. main) duty is towards your own patients and clients. So, if for example, you work in a hospital you have more weighty obligations towards patients on your own wards. Nevertheless you also have obligations, albeit weaker ones, towards patients on neighbouring wards (Edwards 1996). This means that if you became aware of, say, gross malpractice on a neighbouring ward, you would have to do something about it (for example, report it to your line manager).

According to most codes of professional conduct the duty to act beneficently extends even further – to include not just your colleagues, patients and clients and their relatives but also the general public. However, you have obligations to yourselves too and your dependants. To put this another way: you are not obliged to benefit others if to do so would seriously harm your own moral interests (Johnstone 1999).

In summary, then, the principle of beneficence is potentially very broad in that it can be said to generate obligations to all those who may be affected, directly or indirectly, by your conduct.

●━πτ *Keywords*

Non-maleficence

Acting in such a manner as to avoid causing harm (e.g. pain and suffering) to patients

Non-maleficence

Put simply, **non-maleficence** means that you have a duty not to harm others nor subject them to risk of harm (Rumbold 1999). Non-maleficence is commonly described as less morally demanding than beneficence because it generates fewer obligations. Most importantly it does not usually require positive action. What this means is that generally you do not have be a Good Samaritan – i.e. to help strangers in distress. Nevertheless, the moral requirement not to harm or injure others is more complex than it first appears. This is because we can define 'harm' in a variety of ways. How the harm is caused may also be problematic in practice.

Defining 'harm'

Harm can be physical and so include pain, disability, discomfort and death. But it can also be psychological and thus cover mental distress, humiliation, exploitation, even annoyance and so forth. According to Beauchamp and Childress (2001, p. 116) harm should be defined broadly as: thwarting, defeating or setting back some party's interests (interests being all those things in which one has a stake).

But whether a broad or narrow definition of harm is adopted, it is not a neutral, value-free concept. In other words, like the concept of benefit, it is a subjective term – what counts as a harm to one person may not be a harm at all to another.

How can 'harm' be caused?

Harm can be caused deliberately – resulting from, say, abuse, assault or exploitation. But a person can also harm another (or put them at risk) without any malicious or harmful intent (i.e. it can be unintentional). In health-care contexts unintentional harm is likely to be caused by careless or negligent care or treatment. But, as with deliberate harm, unintentional harm can have both trivial and serious consequences.

Because harm can be interpreted broadly it can also be caused by intimidation, inappropriate pressure or undue influence. Misleading or misinforming patients about the risks associated with a particular procedure so that they accept treatment they would otherwise refuse can thus be a form of harm.

In summary, therefore, harm can be caused in a wide variety of ways, ranging from the intentional to the unintentional. Finally it is worth noting that it is possible to harm someone even though you set out to benefit that person. That this is possible, i.e. that a 'good' act can have a 'bad' outcome, raises questions about the relationship between the principles of non-maleficence and beneficence. Are they, as many suggest, just two sides of the same coin?

The relationship between non-maleficence and beneficence

The reason why some philosophers join beneficence and non-maleficence together as a single principle is because almost every nursing, medical or other 'health' intervention that aims to benefit patients may at the same time also harm them. As Rumbold observes (1999, p. 222) sometimes the harm will be unavoidable, even intentional. But at other times it can be unintentional and unexpected. For example, surgery may restore health but it can also carry risks. Similarly, drugs may cure but can have side-effects.

It is perhaps obvious, then, that you should think about the principles of beneficence and non-maleficence at the same time. In other words, benefits and harms need always to be balanced against each other. From this balancing exercise – the outcome of which will depend on each person's evaluation of what is harmful and good for them – should emerge what is the morally 'right' course of action. Or, to put it another way, that which will cause the least harm and the most good.

Top tips

- Rules of non-maleficence usually begin with 'do not'
- There are limits to the principle of beneficence; in particular you are not obliged to act beneficently if doing so would seriously harm your own significant moral interests
- Balancing benefit and harm means making sure that the risks are never worse than the benefits gained

Key points

- The principle of beneficence requires you to act in ways that promote the well-being of others
- The principle of non-maleficence means you must not harm patients but it does not require you to act as a Good Samaritan, i.e. to help strangers in distress

Responsibility and accountability – moral and professional aspects

Although the principles of beneficence and non-maleficence provide the moral foundations for the various obligations in your code of professional conduct they are unlikely to be very useful in giving you much practical guidance about how to solve a particular problem or dilemma. For more practical guidance on what is expected of you we must therefore look elsewhere, in particular to the concepts of responsibility and accountability. As we shall see, these concepts are closely connected and in some ways overlap – which explains why they are so often used interchangeably. But they do not mean the same thing. We shall deal with each separately.

Responsibility

Responsibility is a term that can be understood in several different ways. If we think about **moral responsibility**, for example, we are talking about a person's free will and freedom to use his/her judgement as s/he sees fit. On the other hand **professional responsibility** refers to the special skills and expertise you have acquired as a member of your profession. Most importantly, the idea of professional responsibility sends out a strong message to the public that you have reached a reasonable level of competence and trustworthiness. In other words, you have the skills and expert knowledge that bear directly on the well-being of others.

Finally there is legal responsibility. As we shall see below, this is reflected in the law of negligence. But whether the focus is on moral, professional or legal responsibility the two aspects of responsibility which are most relevant in health care are:

- **Causal responsibility**: have you caused something to happen?
- **Role responsibility**: what is your job?

Causal responsibility – have you caused something to happen?

Causal responsibility basically means that you have caused something to happen (or produced something). It generally refers to consequences, results and outcomes and includes both actions and omissions (failing to act). Suppose, for example, you forget to give a patient pain relief. In such a situation it is relatively easy to claim that you have caused that patient harm. But in some cases it might not be so easy to link what you have done (or have not done) with the harm that a patient has suffered. You may have been working as

Keywords

Moral responsibility
Accepting and carrying the burden of judgement and decision in matters of right and wrong

Keywords

Professional responsibility
The responsibility that arises from mastery of a special body of advanced knowledge that 'professionals' possess

part of a team, for example, another member of which may also have been negligent. So there may have been several 'causes' of the patient's injuries. Or the procedure may have been very complex and technical, making it difficult to establish exactly what went wrong and who was responsible.

As we shall see below, proving negligence (i.e. that someone is legally responsible) in this kind of case can be very difficult, if not impossible. Yet morally (and professionally) you are clearly responsible.

Note too that it is not only human beings who can cause something to happen, since conditions (e.g. staff shortages, poor equipment, inadequate resources and so forth) may also cause accidents or result in a patient being injured or harmed in some way.

Role responsibility – what is your job?

You are responsible for something in this sense if it is your job (or task) to deal with it (Downie and Calman 1994, p. 80). The focus here is therefore on your particular role or, to put it another way, what you are employed to do in your contract of employment. This type of responsibility is very flexible because different roles or jobs bring with them different responsibilities. So, although we can say that, at very general level, all health professionals have four basic fundamental responsibilities – to promote health, prevent illness, restore health and alleviate suffering – the way these basic responsibilities will be carried out can vary enormously. Thus if you work in an intensive care unit your daily responsibilities are likely to differ from those of a nurse working in the community or in primary care. And what happens if you learn new or additional skills? Will your 'role responsibility' change?

Extending your role – 'advanced' practice

Learning new skills – so called advanced practice – was officially outlined in the policy document *Making a Difference* (Department of Health 1999). Yet well before then nurses had increasingly taken over a variety of responsibilities that had previously been undertaken by doctors. This development has been described in a number of ways (i.e. as nurse-led care, extended roles and enhanced roles). But whatever the name used there can be no doubt that nurses now undertake a much wider range of clinical tasks than they did in the past. That they will continue to do so is also beyond doubt since the NHS plan (2000) identified 10 new key roles for nurses, e.g. referrals, admitting and discharging patients, diagnostic testing and prescribing, performing minor surgery, setting up (and running) nurse-led clinics (e.g. dermatology). Other areas where nurses have expanded their roles include NHS Direct and Walk-in Centres.

While these changes have helped break down some of the barriers between medicine and nursing, they do raise important ethical questions. As Burnard and Chapman ask (2003, p. 60), do they mean that traditional nursing tasks should now be carried out by unregistered staff such as health-care assistants? If so, where should ultimate responsibility lie if something goes wrong? And what if you are asked to do something you have not been trained to do? It is important to remember, in short, that your role is not just about performing particular tasks but also about issues such as competence, and maintaining and improving professional knowledge.

Reflective activity

- Think about ways in which you could extend your role.
- Think about what your code of professional conduct says about taking responsibility for tasks beyond your competence.

Key points   Top tips

- 'Being responsible' can mean a) that it is your job or role to deal with something and/or b) that you have caused something to happen
- Extending your role means that your responsibility has increased

Accountability

In recent years discussion about the nature and scope of accountability has become widespread. This is largely due to the assumption that accountability will reduce errors and therefore the number of negligence claims (Harpwood 2001). The Health Act 1999 has further reinforced this emphasis by formalising the 'culture of accountability' both by setting up new structures (such as NICE) and by introducing clinical governance (see Chapter 2). Systems have also been put in place to make sure that blame-free error reporting becomes the norm. But, as with the concept of responsibility, there are several types of accountability, i.e. you can be morally, professional and legally accountable. Before looking at these various aspects of accountability, however, it is important to distinguish accountability from responsibility (with which it is often confused).

Thus you can be responsible for something – in the sense that you caused it to happen – without being accountable. Suppose you make a mistake and harm a patient because responsibility has been inappropriately delegated to you (despite your protests that you were not competent). In this kind of situation you would almost certainly not have to account for your actions. Instead, accountability would rest with the person who should have ensured that you were properly clinically supervised.

Put very simply, therefore, **accountability** is about justifying your actions or omissions and establishing whether there are good enough reasons for acting in the way you did. As Wallace states (2002. p. 9) being personally accountable means you are expected to justify your actions on the grounds of best practice and knowledge, informed by good clinical judgement.

We shall now turn to the different types of accountability. As we shall see below, the law of negligence governs legal accountability, i.e. the extent to which you can be held liable in law for your actions. Moral accountability is very similar but does not necessarily overlap with the legal model. Indeed, the two can come into conflict. Consider this example: a patient's prescription for pain relief is too low (so she is in severe pain). If you ignore the prescription and top it up you will have to account for your actions legally – since you have overstepped the prescription. Morally, however, by relieving a patient's pain you may feel you have done the right thing – and so can justify your actions.

Another kind of accountability is professional accountability. Broadly this means complying with your code of professional conduct. Yet as we noted above, your code is not designed to provide comprehensive answers to all the situations you will face in practice. Furthermore, even if you follow your code you cannot always assume that your actions are therefore morally right too. In other words, professional and moral accountability do not in practice necessarily coincide (Hendrick 2000, pp. 62–66).

Keywords

Accountability
Being required to answer for your actions, explaining why something was (or was not) done

Reflective activity

Think of a situation in which you could justify your actions 'professionally' but not morally.
Think about what your code says about your personal accountability.

Legal responsibility and accountability

This section discusses when you can be held legally responsible and accountable. There are several channels of accountability, but the main focus will be on the tort system, namely negligence law – the most common action in health contexts for NHS patients seeking compensation. Because it is only very exceptionally that health professionals face criminal prosecutions, the role of the criminal law will not be considered here (for an account of criminal negligence see Mason *et al.* 2002, pp. 305–308). Similarly, limited space prevents a discussion of NHS complaints procedures (on which see Montgomery 2003, pp. 112–122).

The law of negligence

In this introduction we look at two issues:

- The rise in negligence claims
- The functions of negligence law.

The rise in negligence claims

There can be little doubt that there has been a very sharp rise in the money spent on litigation (litigation is the term used for negligence claims) since the 1970s – rising from £1 million in 1974 (approx. £6.33 million at 2002 prices) to £446 million in 2002. Such a huge rise might suggest that there is a malpractice crisis but the figures are difficult to interpret accurately, not least because it was not until the 1990s that the NHS began to keep official records of medical accidents. The amount paid in compensation is also much higher now than in the past – which may distort the picture further. Yet, however difficult the figures are to interpret, claims against health professionals have certainly risen very sharply. How can this increase be explained?

No single factor is to blame but, with an estimated 50 million clinical decisions now being taken (for every million of the population every year), it is perhaps not surprising that there are 'adverse outcomes of care' (Department of Health 2003). Explanations for the rise in claims are summarised in the box below.

Reasons for rise in negligence claims

- **The nature of modern medicine**. Advances in medical technology, greater complexity of diagnostic and therapeutic procedures, 'miracle' drugs and so forth all increase the opportunities for things to go wrong
- **Increased patient expectation**. Changing attitudes to illness and health encourage 'empowered' patients not just to seek treatment for conditions once seen as untreatable but also to expect cures
- **Changed attitudes to life's misfortunes**. The so-called 'compensation' culture makes patients less tolerant of errors and thus more insistent that they should be compensated
- **The consumer society**. Emphasis on patients as consumers of health (in which health care is seen as a competitive business), coupled with the media's eagerness to disclose mistakes, encourages patients to assert their 'rights' to complain
- **Deterioration of the relationship between patients and health professionals**. Greater access to medical records and public interest in various scandals have led to increased distrust of the assumed skill and honour of professionals

Functions of negligence law

Although the vast majority of negligence claims never come to trial (95% are settled out of court), it remains a popular action. This is despite the fact that problems with negligence actions are well documented (see below for reform proposals). Much of the continuing appeal of negligence actions lies in the functions the law is said to fulfil. These are outlined in the box below.

Functions of negligence law

- **Compensation**. This is the main function – damages awarded are intended to put victims in the position they would have been if they had not been injured; compensation can include lost earning potential, higher living expenses, cost of long-term care
- **Deterrence**. Legal action and its impact on professional reputations is thought to promote good practice and encourage practitioners to maintain high standards
- **Retribution**. Injured patients may see tort action as a form of revenge, i.e. punishment for the wrong they have suffered
- **Investigation**. Litigation may be the only way to prompt an explanation and, ultimately, an apology for what happened

Basic elements in negligence

To win a negligence case claimants (the name for those suing for compensation) must prove three things. These are:

- That a duty of care was owed, i.e. the defendant was responsible for the victim's care
- That the defendant breached that duty, i.e. the defendant failed to reach the standard of practice required by law
- That damage (that the law recognises) ensued, i.e. the injuries suffered were caused by that failure.

Duty of care: who are you responsible for?

In most health-care situations it is fairly easy to establish that a duty of care exists and it is rarely a matter of dispute. This is because a duty is owed whenever a practitioner has assumed responsibility for someone, i.e. has undertaken to use his/her skills for that person. Accordingly, you will owe a duty not only to patients and clients on your ward (or on your list) but also to those you are caring for or treating in other settings – such as specialist clinics (e.g. family planning clinics), outpatient departments, A&E, the community and so forth.

In some situations, however, the existence of a duty is less obvious. Consider, for example, your legal responsibility for the following:

- Patients who refuse to leave hospital
- Patients who wish to discharge themselves
- Victims of accidents you come across when off duty
- A women who goes into labour in a public place
- Patients' relatives, carers and visitors.

To find out to whether you owe a duty in these (and other) situations you need to apply the modern **'neighbour'** test. Applying this test (see *Caparo Industries* v. *Dickman* [1990]) means that you could (in theory) owe a duty of care to a potentially very wide group of people. In practice, however, the courts have been reluctant to extend legal responsibility beyond the ordinary health professional–patient relationship (and have in fact defined that relationship very narrowly).

So far we have looked at your personal legal responsibility. In some situations, however, a duty of care is owed by hospitals themselves. Called **direct liability**, this type of duty of care requires hospitals, and other provider units, to provide 'a reasonable regime

Keywords
....

Neighbour test
Establishes when a duty of care exists, i.e. whenever a) the damage is foreseeable, b) there is a sufficiently 'proximate' (near) relationship between the claimant and the defendant and c) it is just, fair and reasonable to impose a duty

Keywords
....

Direct liability
A claim based on this type of duty alleges that a hospital (or other provider unit) has failed to manage its services properly

of care', i.e. a safe system of care. What this means is that the hospital itself may face a negligence claim if a victim is harmed because of, say, defective equipment, inadequate resources, too few suitably qualified and competent staff and so on. Cases to date have imposed direct liability when a trust used negligently drafted consent forms, when no system was in place for checking equipment and when staff were inadequately supervised (Montgomery 2003, p. 182).

Note finally the doctrine of *vicarious liability*. Even if you are negligent it is very unlikely that you will have to bear the cost of any claim yourself. This is because under the doctrine of vicarious liability your employer will be sued instead. In other words, employers are indirectly responsible for the negligent acts or omissions of their employees (clinical and non-clinical), providing the negligence occurred in the course of employment (Dimond 2002).

Key points | **Top tips**

- The neighbour test does not require you to act as a Good Samaritan
- This means you have no legal responsibility to help strangers in distress

---

Key points | Top tips

- The neighbour test establishes when a duty of care is owed
- A duty of care can be owed either by you personally or by hospitals or other provider units

---

Breach of duty: what standard of care does the law require?

Once a duty has been established the next step is to prove that the duty has been breached. The crucial question is, therefore: What standard of care does the law require? A very general reply is that the law expects you to exercise reasonable care and skill in all the tasks you undertake. To find out more about what the phrase 'reasonable standard of care' means we have to refer to the famous case of *Bolam* v. *Friern Hospital Management Committee* (1957). This case, and the standard of care it established, is popularly known as the **Bolam test**.

O━┱ *Keywords*

Bolam test

Refers to the general legal principle that practitioners who have acted in the same way as other reasonably competent members of their profession will not normally be found to have been negligent

The Bolam test

According to the Bolam test health professionals will not be liable in negligence if they have followed 'accepted practice'. What this basically means is that you are judged against standards that are set by your peers, i.e. those doing the same kind of work. So, a specialist nurse (e.g. a neonatal nurse) is judged by the standards of other neonatal nurses. If, therefore, in giving evidence, other professionals working in the same field or speciality as you confirm that your actions come within a range of acceptable practice, the claimant is very unlikely to win his/her claim. In effect, then, the Bolam test allows health professionals to determine the legal standard of care.

Other important aspects of the Bolam test to note are:

- If your role has been extended – e.g. you have more independence in, say, diagnosis or treatment – you are judged by the standards of other reasonably competent practitioners who have taken on the same additional responsibilities as you
- Standards expected are not the highest level of skills, i.e. you only have to show that you have reached the same standard as the ordinary competent practitioner
- The test sets the minimum standard below which you must not fall.

Applying Bolam

The courts have heard several important cases since Bolam – exploring the implications of the case in different kinds of scenarios. Some of the most important questions that have arisen are the following:

What if there are differences of opinion?

Suppose you can carry out a procedure or treatment in a variety of different ways. How is the law to decide which one is 'accepted practice'? The answer is clear. Judges will not choose between competing views and practices. In short, they will not decide which one is best (*Maynard* v. *West Midlands RHA* [1985]). So the fact that you might do something differently from your peers is not necessarily evidence of negligence (providing, of course, you can show that at least some other reasonably competent practitioners would have acted in a similar way to you).

When are standards judged?

The law accepts that standards change as current knowledge and skills develop. Standards are therefore judged at the date of the incident and not at a later date (*Roe* v. *Minister of Health* [1954]).

The law does not, therefore, expect you to have the benefit of hindsight.

How up to date do you have to be?

Journal articles, leading textbooks, guidelines, circulars (from, for example, the NHS Executive) and so on can vary in both their frequency and status – i.e. not all will have yet been absorbed into current accepted practice. How can you read them all? Do you have to? As far as the law is concerned it is now well established that you must keep up to date with all major developments in your own field. In other words the duty to keep up to date is a reasonable one.

So you do not have to know all there is to be known but you should nevertheless be aware of mainstream literature and be familiar with, for example, changes in treatment or procedures that have been widely adopted in your particular field as 'best practice'.

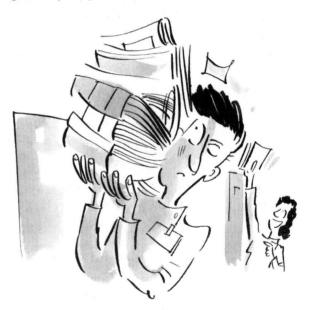

Being aware of current procedures and treatments.

Can you depart from accepted practice?

Suppose, for example, that you decide to use a new and different technique rather than the traditional one. If something goes wrong, will you automatically be found liable? The answer depends on whether departing from conventional practice could be justified, bearing in mind all the circumstances (*Clarke* v. *MacLennan* [1983]). These would include the implications of changing practice and appraisal of new research.

When are breaches most likely to occur?

Typical actions involving nurses have generally concerned allegations that they have not properly supervised patients (see, for example, *Hay* v. *Grampian Health Board* [1995]).

However, negligence can occur in all aspects of care and treatment and in most fields of health care. The most recent data (Department of Health 2003) shows that:

- In NHS hospitals the largest category of claims for negligent care are death and unnecessary pain (accounting for over a fifth of such claims); 10% of hospital inpatient admissions may result in some kind of adverse event

- In primary care over half of claims are for failed or missed diagnosis and almost a quarter for medication errors

- The hospital medical specialities attracting most claims are the various branches of surgery, as well as obstetrics and gynaecology (almost two-thirds of all claims between them)

- Birth-related brain damage (including cerebral palsy) alone accounted for 60% of all annual expenditure on medical litigation in 2002/2003

- Some 5% of the general population report suffering some injury or other adverse effect of medical care; almost a third of those claim that the event had a permanent effect on their health.

Challenging Bolam

In this section we look briefly at challenges to the Bolam test – which has long been criticised for allowing health professionals themselves to set the legal standard of care.

The 'Bolitho' approach

The most important case to challenge Bolam in recent years is *Bolitho* v. *Hackney Health Authority* (1997). The reason why this case provoked so much interest was because all five Law Lords (in the House of Lords) said that: '*the judge, before accepting a body of opinion as being responsible, reasonable or respectable, will need to be satisfied . . . that the experts have weighed up the risks and benefits and have reached a defensible conclusion*'.

This new approach suggested that the courts would be more willing than in the past to question professional opinion – even perhaps setting the standard of care themselves. What seems to have happened in practice, however, is that while the courts may now more often critically scrutinise 'accepted practice' – to ensure that expert opinion is honest, objective and logical – they will only very rarely reject it (Montgomery 2003). In other words, the fundamental principle is that standards will continue to be set by practitioners.

Clinical governance/guidelines

Several commentators (e.g. Harpwood 2001, Montgomery 2003) suggest that clinical governance (see Chapter 2) and **clinical guidelines** could both be used to challenge the Bolam test because they are now key aspects of quality improvement initiatives in the new NHS. As such, they must be taken very seriously. What this means is that if you do not comply with them (suppose, for example, you were not aware of their existence in relation to a particular procedure) it would be much easier than in the past to prove that you had breached the legal standard of care. In short, clinical governance and clinical guidelines have the potential to define the legal standard of care. Or to put it another way, they may be absorbed into the Bolam test and so become the responsible body of professional opinion and 'accepted practice' that you are expected to follow – if it is reasonable to do so. (Dimond 2002, p. 189).

◐━ᴋ *Keywords*

Clinical guidelines

Also referred to as protocols, practice parameters and clinical pathways, these are (like health circulars issued by the NHS Executive) designed to assist practitioner and patient decisions about appropriate health care for specific clinical circumstances, reduce variations in practice and improve efficiency

Top tips

Things you should know about clinical guidelines:
- They can originate from many different sources, e.g. individual departments, hospitals or trusts, national bodies
- The National Institute of Clinical Excellence is a key creator of clinical guidelines
- Whatever their source they are not a substitute for professional judgement

Reflective activity

Think of an incident at work when the standard of care fell below that which was normally required. Why did the incident happen? What procedures were put in place to prevent it happening again?

Key points

- The Bolam test sets the legal standard of care
- The Bolam test means that normally professionals set the standard of care themselves

Causation – how were the claimant's injuries caused?

The last step in a negligence action is to prove that the breach of duty caused (or materially contributed to) the claimant's injury (or harm). In theory, this should not be difficult to establish, for two reasons. First, claimants only have to prove that it was 51% likely that the negligent act caused their injuries. Secondly, the standard 'but for' test can (and often does) work well. According to this test claimants simply need to show that but for the defendant's conduct they would not have been injured. But in practice proving this causal link can be the hardest hurdle to overcome for several reasons:

- **Delay**. Negligence cases typically take years to come to court during which time memories may have faded and important records may have been mislaid.
- **Complexity of scientific evidence**. Some claims, especially for alleged drug-induced injuries and illnesses caused by medical devices are likely to rely on conflicting and very complex epidemiological, immunological and legal evidence (Mason *et al.* 2002, pp. 302–305).
- **Pre-existing medical conditions**. Claimants are usually suffering from an illness or injury. So the fact that their ill health is worse could be due to the natural progression of their original illness or condition (rather than the negligent treatment).
- **Too many possible causes of the injuries**. If the injuries have several possible causes it may be impossible to establish which one was the most legally significant – as in *Wilsher* v. *Essex AHA* (1988), see box below.

Wilsher v. Essex AHA (1988)

Facts

Martin Wilsher was born prematurely suffering from various illnesses, including oxygen deficiency. His prospects of survival were poor and he was placed in a 24-hour special care unit. He was looked after by a medical team consisting of two consultants, a senior registrar, several junior doctors and trained nurses. He needed extra oxygen to survive. An inexperienced doctor mistakenly inserted a catheter into a vein rather than an artery but then asked the senior registrar to check what he had done. The registrar failed to spot the mistake and a few hours later when replacing the catheter did exactly the same thing himself. As a result, Martin was given excess oxygen. Martin claimed the extra oxygen caused his blindness.

continued

Court's decision

The court rejected Martin's claim, even though it accepted that the registrar had been negligent (when he put the catheter into a vein rather than an artery). The reason why Martin lost was this: although excess oxygen could cause blindness there are at least five other possible causes of blindness in premature babies. With so many competing causes, the scientific evidence linking the negligence with the blindness was inconclusive.

But even if claimants can prove causation to get compensation (called damages) they still have to show that their injuries were 'reasonably foreseeable', i.e. that they were not too remote. The kinds of injury that the courts have recognised include:

- Personal injury, pain and suffering
- Death
- Loss of ability to have children
- Post-traumatic shock syndrome
- Loss or damage to property.

Note, however, that compensation may be reduced if claimants are partly at fault – this is called contributory negligence (Dimond 2002, pp. 111–118).

Over to you

Visit www.doh.gov.uk/riskman, then answer these questions:

- What is risk management?
- How effective (in reducing and preventing accidents) have risk management processes been in your practice?

Key points   Top tips

- Causation means that claimants must prove a causal link between a breach of duty and the harm they have suffered
- Compensation cannot be obtained for all forms of 'harm' – only that which the law decides is 'foreseeable'
- Compensation can be reduced if the claimant's own behaviour contributed to his/her injuries

Reform

In this section we discuss the most common criticisms of the law of negligence as a system of paying compensation, and current reform proposals.

Criticisms of current law

The most common criticisms are that the law:

- Is complex
- Is unfair – apparently similar cases may reach different outcomes
- Is slow – cases can take up to 4 years from time of claim to settlement
- Is costly – in legal fees, diversion of clinical staff time from clinical care, staff morale and public confidence
- Fosters a climate of blame, acrimony and confrontation
- Undermines health professional–patient relationships
- Discourages the reporting of errors.

Reform proposals

Proposals for reform were outlined in a report called *Making Amends: A new NHS redress scheme* (Department of Health 2003). The proposed new arrangements would have four main elements:

- An investigation of the incident
- Provision of an explanation
- Development and delivery of a package of care (such as remedial treatment)
- Payments (e.g. for pain and suffering).

Patients would be eligible for payments for serious shortcomings in NHS care if the harm could have been avoided and if the adverse outcome was not the result of natural progression of the illness. Payment would be made up to £30 000 (families of babies suffering brain damage at birth could be eligible for up to £100 000 a year, in addition to other one-off payments, e.g. for home adaptations at various interval throughout the child's life).

Although not a full-blooded no-fault scheme of the sort that the four Nordic nations and New Zealand have, the proposed system has been widely welcomed as an important first step to a 'less confrontational and more efficient system than the present one' (Department of Health 2003).

Top tips

- To view the report (which contains lots of information about the present system) visit www.publications.doh.uk/makingamends/index
- The proposed new scheme would not take away a person's right to sue through the courts

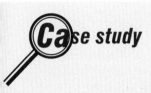

Case study

Learning 'on the job' when resources are scarce

You arrive at work one day to discover that, because two colleagues are off sick with flu, staffing levels are lower than ever before. As the morning progresses, you get more and more worried about the pressure you are under but have no time to do anything about it. Towards the end of your shift you are asked to carry out a procedure that you have watched others do a few times but have never done yourself. Normally you would not be asked – you have only recently qualified and are the most junior member of staff. But given staffing levels you are delegated the task. You are well aware that you lack the experience to take on responsibility for the procedure but because of the staff shortages and your fear of being thought incompetent you go ahead anyway.

Regrettably things go badly wrong and the patient suffers as a result.

Reflective activity

Are you responsible for the patient's injuries? In other words:

1. As a newly qualified practitioner are you expected to reach the same standard as a more experienced, senior member of staff?
2. Can you blame staff shortages for the accident?

---

1. Inexperience

Legal responsibility

It is no defence to claim inexperience. The patient is entitled to receive a reasonable standard of care. If you were in any doubt about your abilities you should at the very least have called for assistance. Then, even if you had made a mistake, the very fact that you had called for help would have been the responsible thing to do (i.e. it would mean that you had satisfied the required standard of care). Accordingly, you would not be personally liable. Put simply, the law allows inexperienced staff to 'learn on the job' but only if they rely on supervision when tackling new or unfamiliar tasks.

Note that the person who delegated the task to you might be legally responsible if s/he knew (or ought to have known) that you were not competent to carry out the task.

Case study continued

Moral and professional responsibility

In failing to acknowledge that you were not competent to carry out the procedure you have not only broken the moral rules of non-maleficence and beneficence but have also breached your code of professional conduct. Accordingly, you may face disciplinary action.

2. Staff shortages

Legal liability

The factors that would be considered in deciding whether you were personally liable include:

- Whether you had informed your manager that, because of pressure of work (caused by staff shortages), you could not provide a reasonable standard of care
- Whether appropriate priorities had been set
- Whether someone should have supervised you
- Whether the incident was reasonably foreseeable
- Whether the procedure could have been postponed.

Depending on your answers to the above, it is of course possible that your employer is also directly liable – for failing to provide a safe working environment by, for instance, not monitoring work levels regularly and not ensuring that there were enough qualified staff to provide a reasonable standard of care. Remember, too, that if you decide to raise your concerns about staffing levels (or any other factors that may jeopardise patient care) you are protected from victimisation under the Public Interest Disclosure Act 1998.

Moral and professional responsibility

If lack of resources jeopardise the provision of safe and appropriate care you should follow your code of professional conduct. This requires you to minimise the risk to patients and clients by reporting your concerns to a senior person. Note that the factors relevant to determining your legal liability (see above) would also be relevant here. Failure to comply with your code means that you have again failed to follow the principles of beneficence and non-maleficence and may also be professionally accountable. Accordingly, you will have to explain your actions – why you did not ask for help, for example.

Reflective activity

What have you learnt from this case study about what you should do when working under pressure?

What would you do if you feared victimisation for 'whistle-blowing'?

The relationship between law and ethics

In this last section we compare the legal and ethical concepts of responsibility and accountability.

Similarities between law and ethics

- **Common vocabulary**. The concept of fault (which suggests moral blameworthiness) underpins terms such as duty of care and reasonableness.
- **Common function**. Setting acceptable standards of acceptable behaviour.
- **Similar outcomes**. Practitioners who failure to reach acceptable standards can be sued and/or face disciplinary action.

Differences between law and ethics

- **Duty of care**. The ethical duty of care is wider than the legal duty. Health professionals may, for example, have a moral and professional duty to help strangers but legally they have no responsibility for them.
- **Standard of care**. The legal standard of care, which aims to set a minimum level of competence below which practitioners must not fall, is lower than the ethical standard, which aims for the best possible level of care.
- **Harm**
  - If causation is not proved there is no legal liability even if a practitioner has breached his/her duty of care. In contrast, a practitioner may be morally and professionally accountable even if no harm occurs.
  - Only certain types of harm can be compensated for in law, i.e. those that are foreseeable. But both morally and professionally practitioners are accountable for all the harm they have caused.

RRRRRapid recap

Check your progress so far by working through each of the following questions.

1. What are the functions of negligence law?
2. Which ethical principles form the moral foundations of your code of professional conduct?
3. What is the difference between responsibility and accountability?
4. What are the elements of a negligence claim?
5. What is the Bolam test?

If you have difficulty with more than one of the questions, read through the section again to refresh your understanding before moving on.

References

Beauchamp, T.L. and Childress, J.F. (2001) *Principles of Biomedical Ethics*, 5th edn. Oxford University Press, Oxford.

Burnard, P. and Chapman, C. (2003) *Professional and Ethical Issues in Nursing*, 3rd edn. Baillière Tindall, Edinburgh.

Department of Health (1999) *Making a Difference: Strengthening the nursing, midwifery and health visiting contribution to healh and health care*. HMSO, London.

Department of Health (2003) *Making Amends: A consultation paper setting out proposals for reforming the approach to clinical negligence in the NHS*. HMSO, London.

Dimond, B. (2002) *Legal Aspects of Nursing*, 3rd edn. Pearson Education, Harlow.

Downie, R.S. and Calman, K.C. (1994) *Health Respect*, 2nd edn. Oxford University Press, Oxford.

Edwards, S.D. (1996) *Nursing Ethics: A principle-based approach*. Macmillan, Basingstoke.

Fry, S. and Johnstone, M.J. (2002) *Ethics in Nursing Practice: A guide to ethical decision making*. Blackwell Science, Oxford.

Harpwood, V. (2001) *Negligence in Health Care: Clinical claims and risk in context*. Informa, London.

Hendrick, J. (2000) *Law and Ethics in Nursing and Health Care*. Stanley Thornes, Cheltenham.

Johnstone, M.J. (1999) *Bioethics: A nursing perspective*, 3rd edn. Saunders, Marrickville, NSW.

Mason, J.K., McCall Smith, R.A. and Laurie, G.T. (2002) *Law and Medical Ethics*, 6th edn. Butterworths, London.

Montgomery, J. (2003) *Health Care Law*. Oxford University Press, Oxford.

Rumbold, G. (1999) *Ethics in Nursing Practice*, 3rd edn. Baillière Tindall, London.

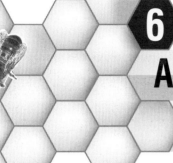

6

Autonomy and consent to treatment

Learning outcomes

By the end of this chapter you should be able to:

- Discuss the principle of autonomy and its practical implications
- Consider the role of paternalism
- Describe the legal principles that underpin the law of consent
- Identify the legal exceptions to the principle of consent.

Introduction

Respect for a person's autonomy and the right to consent to or refuse treatment are now widely accepted as central values in health care that few would openly challenge. Indeed, the idea that individuals have the right to decide whether to undergo treatment reflects one of the most fundamental changes in the relationship between health professionals and patients to have taken place in the last 30 years. This chapter explores why 'autonomy' has become such a buzz word and what it means to be an autonomous person. The kinds of thing you need to do to make sure you respect your patients' autonomy in practice are also discussed. As you will see, this involves exploring in what circumstances you can make decisions on the patient's behalf, i.e. act paternalistically. As regards the law, we focus on the legal elements of valid consent for adult patients (i.e. those over 18). The chapter concludes with an outline of the legal exceptions to the principle of consent.

Autonomy

Definitions

What is autonomy?

The word **autonomy** comes from the Greek: *autos* (self) and *nomos* ('rule' or 'law'). The word autonomy is commonly defined very broadly as 'self-determination', self-rule, 'being your own person' (Parker and Dickenson 2001, p. 136). Other definitions associate autonomy with the idea of moral reflection, i.e. choosing your own moral position and accepting responsibility for the kind of person you are (Dworkin 1988). Sometimes, too, autonomy is equated with integrity, dignity, independence and identified with qualities such as self-assertion and critical reflection.

Keywords

Autonomy

The capacity to make reasoned decisions, i.e. the ability to think for oneself, to make decisions for oneself and to act on the basis of such thought

○━┓ *Keywords*

Respect for autonomy
Acknowledging a person's
right to hold views, make
choices and take actions
based on personal values and
beliefs

○━┓ *Keywords*

Autonomous person
An individual who runs his/her
own life according to his/her
own values and aspirations

What is respect for autonomy?

In health care ethics, however, it is the principle of **respect for autonomy** to which writers most often refer (see, for example, Beauchamp and Childress 2001). Respect for autonomy basically means treating patients as persons with rights and not as objects of care. What this mainly involves in this context is discussing proposed treatment or care with patients in an open and honest way, allowing them to make their own decisions about what should happen to their bodies and, if they are competent, accepting their choices (Hendrick 2000, p. 31).

What is an autonomous person?

An autonomous person is someone who can write the story of their own life (i.e. live out their 'life plan'). Basically, being autonomous means that you can do whatever it is that you want to do with your life. It generally involves the following:

- **The ability to evaluate/deliberate**. To make a life plan you need to be able to decide for yourself what your personal goals are – goals based on your own freely chosen beliefs and values (Burkhardt and Nathaniel 2002, p. 42).

- **Evaluations must be rational**. Your evaluations (i.e. your decisions and actions) must reflect your life plan. The word 'rational' in this context also means that you do not automatically act on your desires and values. Instead you must consider how far they will enable you to achieve your goals and are in your best interests (Parker and Dickenson 2001, p. 282).

- **The capacity to make decisions**. This means the ability to understand facts; to deliberate on the various options (i.e. grasp the connection between alternative treatments and their effects); to think logically; to imagine situations and feelings; and to relate all these to the making of the decision.

- **The freedom to act**. An autonomous person must have the freedom to act upon his/her choices. This explains why people who are competent – and can thus understand the options available to them and make decisions based on them – are nevertheless said to lack (or have limited) autonomy if they are unable to actually carry through their life plans (Burkhardt and Nathaniel 2002).

The importance of autonomy

As an ethical concept, autonomy is undoubtedly one of the most important concepts in modern moral and political philosophy.

But why has it become so influential? There are three main reasons:

- Western society has traditionally placed great emphasis on the moral importance of freedom (or liberty) for the individual. Indeed, the three most influential political philosophers of the late 20th century – John Rawls, Ronald Dworkin and Joseph Raz – not only saw autonomy as crucial for individual flourishing but also as a key component of the 'good society'.

- The political and cultural climate of the late 20th century – with its emphasis on personal endeavour and initiative as well as individual human rights – has transformed not only the way we see ourselves but also how we relate to other people. Thus sociologists, such as Giddens (1992), have argued that the newly important place of the individual in society means that the autonomous, free-willed, self-reflective person is now the ideal we all aspire to. Or, as Farsides puts it (2002, p. 123), *'to be autonomous is to fit into the picture of what it means to be an effective and successful member of society'*.

- The relationship between health professionals and patients is much more equal and patient-centred than it was in the past. Often now described as a contractual relationship – with each party having rights and duties – it is not surprising that patients, like any other consumers, expect to have their choices respected.

⌇ *Over to you*

Read your code of professional conduct. What does it say about respecting patients' autonomy?

Key points Top tips

- The principle of autonomy implies that people have the freedom to decide how to run their lives
- Being autonomous means having the ability to: a) determine your personal goals; b) understand available options and their consequences; c) decide on a plan of action; and d) act on your choices

---

How to respect patients' autonomy

In health-care situations it is now taken for granted that one of the main ways patients exercise autonomy is through the concept of consent (or informed consent as it is often called). As Chadwick and

Tadd (1992, p. 66) explain: '*the link between consent and autonomy is that, since mature adults are presumed to have the capacity for autonomy, there is a moral requirement to show respect for this autonomy, and part of such respect for autonomy implies, in practical terms, not interfering with people without their consent*'.

But how exactly can you make sure you respect autonomy (and obtain consent) in practice? In other words what obligations does it impose on you? The following are widely accepted as the essential elements of consent:

Communication

Effective communication is not only important as a means of discovering or conveying information but is also acknowledged as the single most important way of securing your patients' co-operation and compliance, i.e. their willingness to participate in treatment. Communication involves listening to patients and talking to them in a language that is familiar to them and is jargon-free (Rumbold 1999). It also involves being sensitive to and respecting cultural differences, i.e. the beliefs, values and practices of different groups in society (Farsides 2002).

> ### Over to you
>
> Read Burnard and Chapman 2003, Appendix 2. Consider what the authors say about the dos and don'ts relating to various cultures.

Truthfulness

At its very simplest the obligation to tell the truth (or the 'duty of veracity' as it is sometimes called) means that you should be honest with patients, i.e. not lie to or deceive them. That patients have the right to be told the truth – especially when they ask specific questions – is now widely accepted as a universal virtue and promoted in all professional codes. But truthfulness describes much more than simply passing on accurate information. Rather it reflects an attitude towards another person that aims to create open and mutually respectful communication (Campbell *et al.* 2001).

> ### Reflective activity
>
> Will telling the truth always benefit your patients?
> Think about a situation from your practice when the truth may be harmful.

Voluntariness

Voluntariness means making decisions freely. According to Beauchamp and Childress (2001, p. 93) a person acts voluntarily 'if he or she wills the action without being under the control of another's influence'. This means that patients should not be coerced (i.e. forced) into accepting treatment they do not want. Nor should they be manipulated, for example by having information withheld from them. More problematic in this context is another form of influence – persuasion. While some persuasion may be acceptable – if it fosters understanding, discussion and rational decision-making – the line between acceptable forms of persuasion and manipulation may be difficult to draw in practice.

Giving information

If patients are not given accurate information they cannot make meaningful and rational choices. So what information should be disclosed? According to Beauchamp and Childress (2001, p. 80) you have a moral obligation to disclose:

- Those facts or descriptions that patients usually consider material in deciding whether to refuse or consent to the proposed intervention
- Information that you as a professional believe to be material
- Your professional recommendations
- The purpose of seeking consent.

The most controversial aspect of giving patients information centres on what risks you have to disclose. Should every risk, however remote or trivial, be disclosed? As we shall see below, these are the kinds of question that have long troubled the courts. But as a moral matter it has been suggested that you should disclose whatever information a reasonable person would want to know, plus whatever else the actual individual wants to know (Brock 1993, p. 50).

Accepting patients' preferences

Respecting your patients' autonomy means accepting their choices, i.e. their right to decide whether or not to undergo any health-care intervention, whatever the outcome. Accordingly you must respect a competent adult's refusal of treatment – even if that refusal may result in harm or death to themselves (or a foetus) unless a court orders otherwise.

Respecting autonomy also means that, providing patients have good reasons, they can act autonomously even when they ask someone else to make a decision for them. Indeed, some patients may refuse to be given any information at all. So what counts as a good reason? According to Hope *et al.* (2003, p. 35) they are that the patient:

- Trusts the health professional's judgement
- Finds making choices about his/her own health difficult
- Believes that the health professional's experience will enable him/her to correctly predict the patient's own response.

Key points | **Top tips**

Respecting autonomy means you must:

- Effectively communicate with patients
- Be truthful
- Enable patients to make decisions freely
- Provide appropriate information
- Accept your patient's preferences

Reflective activity

Do you think patient autonomy has gone too far?

Must you always respect patient autonomy?

In this section we look at the kinds of thing that can impair (or limit) a person's autonomy and what you should do if this happens. Or, to put it another way, we discuss the fact that autonomy is not an absolute principle.

Reasons for limited autonomy – patients who are not autonomous

Some patients, such as newborn babies, very young children and patients (whether children or adults) who are unconscious, are not autonomous because they are unable either to make or to communicate their decisions. As such, there is no doubt that their autonomy is limited. But in other situations a patient's autonomy may be limited because of serious doubts about whether s/he is competent. As we shall see in subsequent chapters, concerns about capacity typically arise in respect of children and adolescents (Chapter 12), elderly people (Chapter 13) and those with mental ill health and/or learning disabilities (Chapter 11). Finally, there are those patients whose ability to make decisions is impaired because of short-term factors such as sedative medicine, pain, anger, stress, fear, drug addiction and so on. Long-term illnesses (physical or mental) can also affect a person's ability to act autonomously. So what happens when autonomy is impaired?

Impact of impaired autonomy – paternalism

When autonomy is impaired patients are either not involved at all (or are involved only minimally) in the decision-making process or alternatively their choices are overridden or disregarded altogether. The moral justification for acting without consent are the principles of beneficence (the duty to do good) and non-maleficence (the duty to do no harm) (Chapter 5). When you apply these principles in practice – i.e. you make decisions about a patient's care or treatment irrespective of their wishes or judgements (or without consulting them at all) – we say you are acting paternalistically.

Paternalism is a complex concept and can be understood in several ways, e.g. in attitudes, language and treatment decisions. Briefly, however, in whatever way it is described it basically involves overriding someone's autonomy because you think it is for their own good (Chadwick and Tadd 1992, p. 188). In the past, paternalism was very common in health care and patients were routinely treated without adequate explanation of what was involved (Mason *et al.* 2002, p. 9). But now paternalistic practice is far less acceptable. This means that if you make a decision for someone without consulting them (or if you ignore their wishes) you must have a very good reason. So what counts as a good enough reason?

Justification for paternalism – good reasons for acting paternalistically

Although what counts as good reason will ultimately depend on the circumstances of each particular case, the following conditions are commonly put forward to justify paternalistic intervention:

- The patient is at risk of significant, preventable harm
- The paternalistic action will probably prevent the harm
- The patient's capacity for rational reflection is either absent or significantly impaired
- At a later time it can be assumed that the patient will approve of the decision taken on his/her behalf
- The benefits to the patient of intervention outweigh the risks.

It should be noted that all these justifications have been debated (e.g. Edwards 1996). What is nevertheless beyond doubt is that

Keywords

Paternalism
Basically, acting or choosing on someone else's behalf without their specific consent or knowledge because you believe it is in their best interests

paternalistic practices are much less likely to be tolerated now than they were in the past.

> ~~Key points~~ **Top tips**
>
> When considering whether a patient's autonomy is limited remember to:
> - Never make assumptions about their competence
> - Accept that patients will have their own views about what is best for them

> **Key points** ~~Top tips~~
>
> - Patients' autonomy may be impaired because they lack (or have limited) capacity
> - Paternalism means making decisions on behalf of patients without their full consent or knowledge

The law of consent

Introduction

The legal principles that underpin the law of consent were first recognised almost 100 years ago in a famous 1914 American case (*Schloendorff* v. *Society of New York Hospitals*), when the judge said: '*Every human being of adult years and sound mind has the right to determine what shall be done with his own body*'.

Since then the courts have repeatedly confirmed that the law takes the right of adults to consent to any touching of their bodies very seriously. This means that, if you do not get your patients' consent or permission before you start any treatment, investigation or care (that involves touching them), you may be liable to legal action. Nor does it make any difference how trivial the procedure is, since the law applies to all physical interventions – from major surgery and the administration or prescription of drugs to assistance with dressing.

Given the seriousness the law attaches to consent, it is not surprising that some of the issues it raises are very complex. What follows is therefore only an outline of those aspects you need to know for everyday practice. Note too that the law relating to children, the elderly and those with mental health and learning disabilities is dealt with in later chapters.

Functions of the law of consent

Consent law is said to perform two different functions. These are:

- **Clinical function**. This aims to foster patients' trust, co-operation and confidence and can involve lengthy counselling and discussions of, for example, the side effects of treatment (see below).
- **Legal function**. This aims to protect health professionals who touch patients from criminal charges and civil claims.

Your role in the consent process

Your legal role in the consent process ultimately depends on your particular responsibilities. These will determine whether you are a primary carer or an advocate.

O─π *Keywords*

Primary carer

Refers to the person who is primarily responsible for the care of a patient

O─π *Keywords*

Advocate

The advocate role of health professionals requires them to act ethically so as to protect patients from harm

- You are the **primary carer** when you are directly responsible for providing treatment – giving an injection, taking a blood sample and so on. Similarly, if you are washing, dressing or feeding patients then it will similarly be your job to obtain consent. Usually it is the individual performing a procedure who has the task of obtaining consent. In certain circumstances, however, you may seek consent on behalf of a colleague if you have been specifically trained for that specific area of practice (NMC 2002).

- You are an **advocate** for the patient when you are not the primary carer but are expected to take an active part in the consent process – advising and counselling patients who may, for example, be uncertain or confused (Rumbold 1999).

> ### Over to you
>
> Read Fry and Johnstone 2002, pp. 37–38. How do the authors define the role of an advocate?

Forms of consent

Only exceptionally – such as in mental health settings, abortion and infertility treatment – does the law lay down rules about what form consent should take. In all other cases the law is silent. This means that consent can either be express/explicit (either written or by word of mouth) or implied (see the box below). All are equally valid.

Forms of consent

Express/explicit

- **Written**. It is standard practice in the NHS to use model forms covering most forms of treatment or other invasive procedures; once signed by a patient these forms provide the best evidence that consent was actually given (unless it is clear that the patient did not understand what s/he was signing).
- **Word of mouth**. Oral consent is typically given for routine, less risky procedures. Widely used in everyday practice it is nevertheless less reliable as a form of consent, being harder to prove later on.

Implied

- **Actions/behaviour**. No words are used and no forms are signed; rather consent is implied when a patient, for example, nods his/her head, rolls up his/her sleeve or opens his/her mouth. This form of consent is the weakest.

Key points **Top tips**

- You can download model consent forms and comprehensive guidance about the law of consent from the Department of Health website: www.doh.gov.uk/consent
- Other helpful information about he law is provided in health circular HSC 2001/023 (Department of Health 2001)

When is consent legally valid?

Whatever form consent takes it is only legally valid (i.e. 'real') if three essential criteria are met. These are that the patient:

- Is acting under his/her own free will (i.e. consent must be voluntary)
- Knows in broad terms what s/he is consenting to (i.e. has received enough information to make a decision)
- Is competent (i.e. able to give consent).

Each of these three elements will be looked at separately.

Voluntariness

Consent is voluntary or free when it is given without pressure, force, manipulation or undue influence. In practice, whether or not consent is free will depend on several factors, including the effect of pain, tiredness, drugs and so on. The institutional setting and the relationship of the 'persuader' to the patient may also be important, especially if s/he is a parent. This aspect of consent was highlighted in the important case of *Re T.* (1992) (see box below).

Re T (1992) – guidance on 'free' consent

Facts

A 20-year-old woman injured in a car accident when she was 34 weeks pregnant was rushed to hospital for an emergency caesarean. Her baby was stillborn. Shortly afterwards she developed an abscess on her lungs but refused treatment on religious grounds. The hospital sought a court order to override her refusal. The issue before the court was whether her mother – a devout Jehovah's Witness – had exerted undue (i.e. too strong an) influence during the time she spent with her soon after she was first admitted.

Court's decision

The Court of Appeal held that T's refusal was not 'free' as she had been under the strong influence of her mother. Accordingly treatment that was in her best interests could be carried out. As the court put it, the real question is: Does the patient really mean what he says or is he merely saying it for a quiet life or to satisfy someone else or because the advice and persuasion to which he has been subjected is such that he can no longer think and decide for himself?

Providing 'enough' information

The issue of how much information the law requires you to give patients (i.e. the legal standard of disclosure) has long been a controversial one. In this section we will look at:

- The two different approaches that can be taken on this issue
- The current approach taken by the courts.

Two possible approaches

- **'Patient' standard.** Requires health professionals to disclose broadly what an average 'reasonable' patient (with that particular illness or condition) would want to know.
- **'Professional' standard.** This allows health professionals to set their own standards of disclosure – although in deciding what to disclose they do have to follow accepted (i.e. responsible) practice. In short, the Bolam test applies (see Chapter 5).

Because the patient standard normally requires more information to be disclosed than the professional standard it is often referred to as 'informed consent' approach. Traditionally, the patient approach has not been favoured by English courts (in contrast to several other countries such as Australia, Canada and the USA). But there are signs that this may be changing as, in more and more cases (e.g. *Smith* v. *Tunbridge Wells HA* [1994]; *Pearce* v. *United Bristol Health Care Trust* [1999]; *Chester* v. *Afshar* [2003]), the courts have found health professionals negligent for failing to give enough information to patients to enable them make a balanced judgement. In other words, the courts rejected the professional standard approach in favour of a more patient-centred one.

The current approach taken by the courts

The combined effect of the leading case of *Sidaway* v. *Bethlem Royal Hospital Governors* (1985) (as modified by more recent case law) and current guidance from the Department of Health is that the legal standard of disclosure is as follows.

- Patients must be given enough information to make a balanced judgement, that is be told in broad terms the nature and purpose of the procedure; its likely risks, in particular those that are 'material' or 'significant' risks (i.e. those that would affect the judgement of a reasonable patient); any alternatives to proposed treatment; and the risks incurred by doing nothing.
- Patients who ask direct questions should be answered truthfully. As Lord Woolf said in *Pearce* v. *United Bristol Healthcare NHS Trust* (1999): '*it is clear that if a patient asks a doctor about a risk, then the doctor is required to give an honest answer*'.

That you should answer questions honestly is also emphasised in guidance from the Department of Health accompanying NHS consent forms.

Top tips

- Be aware that if you fail to comply with the legal duty of disclosure you could face a negligence claim
- Realise that the law on information disclosure is complex and only an outline is provided here
- Understand that, under the principle of 'therapeutic privilege', you can legally withhold information that you think will harm the patient (Mason *et al.* 2002, p. 356)

Key points

- Patients who ask direct questions should be answered truthfully
- To give valid consent patients need to understand in broad terms the nature and purpose of the procedure

Is the patient competent?

To give consent patients must be mentally competent (note that words 'capacity' and competence are often used interchangeably). Currently patients are considered competent if they pass the rather vague test laid down in *Re C.* (1994), i.e. that they can:

- Understand and retain relevant information, especially as to the likely consequences of having or not having the treatment in question
- Use and weigh up this information in reaching a decision.

The *Re C.* test is broadly similar to the proposed new test of capacity proposed in the Mental Capacity Bill 2004 (see Chapter 11). Other important legal aspects of the law are outlined in the box below.

Legal aspects of capacity

- The law assumes adults to be competent unless proved otherwise.
- Incapacity can may arise because of psychiatric illness, brain injury, learning disability, dementia, etc.
- A patient's capacity may be temporarily affected by factors such as confusion, shock, pain, etc.; even so, it should not be automatically assumed that s/he is therefore incapable of consenting.
- The graver the consequences of a decision the greater the level of competence required to take the decision.
- Capacity can fluctuate, in which case it is good practice to establish (while a patient has capacity) what his/her views are about treatment that may be necessary during a period of incapacity (note that these views should be recorded).
- Capacity should not be confused with unreasonable, eccentric or unwise decisions, i.e. patients are entitled to make irrational decisions; nevertheless, irrationality may be a symptom or evidence of incompetence.

Key points Top tips

- Adult patients are legally competent if they can understand and weigh up the information they need to make a decision

Refusal of consent

One of the most difficult situations you may face in practice is when patients refuse life-saving treatment or treatment without which their health will be irreparably damaged. In some cases refusal of treatment may lead to death. But whatever the probable outcome of the refusal the law is clear: providing adult patients are competent they have the absolute legal right to refuse treatment irrespective of the consequences of the decision (*Re M B* (1997); *St George's Healthcare NHS Trust* v. *S* [1998]). The most recent case to confirm this fundamental legal right was *Re B* (2002). This case involved a 43-year-old patient who was paralysed from the neck down. She was kept alive by a ventilator but wanted it switched off. Doctors treating her could not bring themselves to disconnect the ventilator and the patient only finally got her wish when she was transferred to another hospital where her wishes were respected.

Over to you

What does your code of professional conduct advise about refusal of treatment?

Key points Top tips

- Competent adult patients have the absolute legal right to refuse treatment whatever the consequences

Exceptions to the principle of consent

In this section we outline certain special scenarios with the exception of children (which are covered in Chapter 12), the elderly (Chapter 13) and the mentally ill (Chapter 11).

Unconscious adult patients – principle of necessity

When faced with an emergency – typically an unconscious patient arriving in the Accident & Emergency Department – you may have to make on-the-spot decisions as to how to treat them. This situation raises the question as to who has the right to consent to treatment on behalf of an incompetent adult. In other words, is proxy consent in respect of adults lawful? Currently the answer is no. English law does not recognise any general doctrine whereby a spouse (or anyone else) can give legally effective consent to medical treatment to be carried out on an adult.

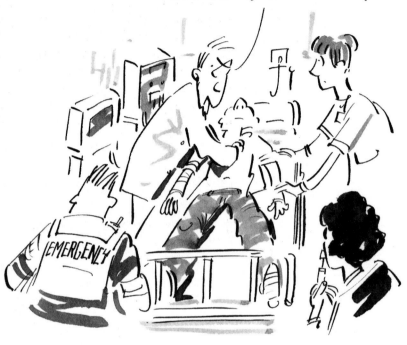

Exceptions to the principle of consent – the incompetent adult.

How then can decisions be made for adults who lack capacity (i.e. are not competent)? It is now well established that the doctrine of necessity covers these situations. According to this doctrine such emergency treatment can be carried out as is necessary to save the patient's life and health (Mason *et al.* 2002; Stauch *et al.* 2002). It is important to remember, however, that you cannot use 'necessity' to take advantage of unconscious patients so as to perform 'non-essential' procedures, i.e. those that are not essential for the patient's survival. The only other limitation on emergency treatment is that the patient might have a 'living will' that prohibits even life-saving surgery (see Chapter 14).

Incompetent adult patients – 'best interests' test

As regards other incompetent adult patients, i.e. those who are not unconscious but who lack the capacity to make their own decisions about treatment, case law has established that any treatment that is in their 'best interests' can be carried out. Treatment covered by the best interests test includes routine procedures as well as major surgery (*Re F* [1990]).

The courts have interpreted the phrase 'best interests' very widely. It includes not just medical interests but also much wider welfare considerations such as the patient's values and preferences (when competent), their psychological health and well-being, quality of life, relationships with family or other carers, spiritual and religious welfare and their own financial interests (*Re M B* [1987]). In acting in the patient's best interests health professionals must, of course, follow the Bolam test (Chapter 5).

Note too that in the vast majority of cases it is not necessary to go to court to get the court's permission before treating incompetent patients. That said, the courts have suggested that it is good practice to seek their approval for the following procedures:

- Sterilisation for contraceptive purposes
- Donation of regenerative tissue such as bone marrow
- Withdrawal of nutrition and hydration from patients in a persistent vegetative state
- Where there is doubt as to the patient's capacity or best interests.

Key points **Top tips**

- Be aware that major changes to the law governing consent to medical treatment in relation to incompetent patients are contained in the draft Mental Capacity Bill 2004
- These changes aim to make it much clearer and easier to make decisions for those who are not able to make their own (see Chapter 11)

Key points Top tips

- Unconscious adult patients can be treated without consent under the doctrine of necessity
- It is lawful to treat incompetent adults without their consent, provided treatment is in their 'best interests'

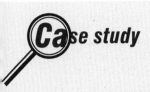

Case study

Jean

Jean is 33 and has two young children. Recently she has been diagnosed with cancer but has refused all treatment even though she knows she will die without it. You are unhappy about Jean's decision, believing that treatment is her only hope, if not of a cure than at least of several more years of life. Moreover, you are convinced that Jean's refusal is at least partly due to the way the various treatment options were explained to her by the doctor. As a consequence you doubt that she has made a free choice. In other words, she might not have refused treatment if she had been adequately informed, i.e. given sufficient information to make an informed decision.

Reflective activity

1. What is your role as patient advocate?
2. If Jean still refuses treatment after she has been given enough information to make a balanced judgement, can her refusal be ignored? Or, to put it another way, does she have the right to make what you think is an 'irrational' decision?

---

1. Advocacy role

Ethical approach

As Tschudin points out (2003), there has been considerable debate surrounding the role of patient advocate. However, if you accept that one part of the advocate's role is to help patients exercise their rights so that they can act autonomously, then there can be little doubt that to perform your role effectively you must ensure that Jean is adequately informed. In other words, you have a moral and professional responsibility to ensure that Jean makes a free choice (Fry and Johnstone 2002). To do this you will have to make sure that she understands the significance of her refusal. This can mean that at the very least you should tell the doctor of your concerns. If this fails to remedy the situation you may decide to provide the information yourself, bearing in mind that the ethical standard of disclosure means that patients are entitled to more information than is required legally (the patient standard).

Legal position

There is no express recognition in English law at present of the role of patient advocate (McHale 2001). That said you do almost certainly have a legal duty to at the very least tell the doctor of your concerns. If your concerns are ignored, the legal position is less clear (unless, of course, you have been given the task of seeking consent on the doctor's behalf, in which case you do have a legal duty to ensure that Jean is adequately informed). Should you provide Jean with the 'missing' information, i.e. in effect refuse to follow the doctor's orders, you may

Case study continued   face disciplinary action (McHale 2001). But, given the emphasis now on openness, honesty and fuller disclosure of information, this is perhaps unlikely. Ultimately, however, your legal responsibility would turn on what your colleagues, i.e. other professionals working in the same field, would have done in this type of situation (i.e. the Bolam test would apply).

2. Refusal of consent

Ethical approach

For Jean's refusal to be respected it must be a decision she is capable of reaching of her own free will. In short, she must be capable of acting autonomously. Jean's capacity is therefore a central issue but in the absence of any obvious physical or psychological factors the assumption must be that she is competent. More problematic is the potential limitation on Jean's autonomy that could arise because of the failure to provide her with sufficient information to make a balanced judgement. For her autonomy to be respected this information must be provided. Only then can she act autonomously. Once this information has been provided, however, then there is no justification for acting paternalistically. In short, Jean's refusal must be accepted.

Legal position

The central legal concerns focus on competence and information disclosure. The law presumes adults are competent – unless there is contrary evidence. And until the Mental Incapacity Bill becomes law the test for capacity is that laid down in *Re C* (1994). According to that test Jean is competent (i.e. she can understand and retain information and can use it to make an informed choice). As to the issue of information, once she has been given enough information to make a balanced judgement, her refusal of treatment, however irrational, must be respected whatever the consequences (*Re B* [2002]). Legally, therefore, you have no right to ignore Jean's refusal and treat her in her 'best interests'.

Reflective activity

What have you learnt from this case study about autonomy?
What obstacles to respecting autonomy does it highlight?

The relationship between law and ethics

Similarities between law and ethics

- **Principle of autonomy**. Both law and ethics are concerned with protecting patients' rights – to make autonomous choices, to self-determination and bodily integrity.

- **'Free' consent**. Both law and ethics are committed to preventing coercion, manipulation and undue pressure.

- **Basic elements**. The same basic elements – competency, voluntariness and sufficient information – are essential to the law of consent and ethics.

- **Making decisions for others**. Both law and ethics have mechanisms for making decisions for those who are incompetent; thus paternalism is justified ethically when patients' autonomy is limited and in law the 'best interest' test applies.

Differences between law and ethics

- **Advocacy**. The moral concept of advocacy is more developed than its legal counterpart, i.e. there is no recognition in law of the role of advocate.

- **Information disclosure.** The ethical standard of disclosure is patient-oriented; as such more detailed information must be provided than the law requires to be disclosed.

- **Truth-telling**. The moral and professional obligation to tell the truth is stronger than the legal one in that health professionals can rely on 'therapeutic privilege' to withhold information they think might harm the patient's health.

RRRRRapid recap

Check your progress so far by working through each of the following questions.

1. What does respect for autonomy mean?
2. Why is autonomy important?
3. What are the essential elements of legal consent?
4. What is the legal consequence of not giving the patient adequate information?
5. How are decisions made for patients who are incompetent?

If you have difficulty with more than one of the questions, read through the section again to refresh your understanding before moving on.

References

Beauchamp, T.L. and Childress, J.F. (2001) *Principles of Biomedical Ethics*, 5th edn. Oxford University Press, Oxford.

Brock, D.W. (1993) *Life and Death: Philosophical essays in biomedical ethics*. Cambridge University Press, Cambridge.

Burkhardt, M.A. and Nathaniel, A.K. (2002) *Ethics and Issues in Contemporary Nursing*, 2nd edn. Delmar, Albany, NY.

Burnard, P. and Chapman, C. (2003) *Professional and Ethical Issues in Nursing*, 3rd edn. Baillière Tindall, Edinburgh.

Campbell, A., Gillett, G. and Jones, G. (2001) *Medical Ethics*, 3rd edn. Oxford University Press, Oxford.

Chadwick, R. and Tadd, W. (1992) *Ethics and Nursing Practice: A case study approach*. Macmillan, Basingstoke.

Department of Health (2001) HSC 2001/023. HMSO, London.

Dworkin, G. (1988) *The Theory and Practice of Autonomy*. Cambridge University Press, Cambridge.

Edwards, S.D. (1996) *Nursing Ethics: A principle-based approach*. Macmillan, Basingstoke.

Farsides, B. (2002) An ethical perspective – consent and patient autonomy. In: *Nursing Law and Ethics*, 2nd edn (eds J. Tingle and A. Cribb). Blackwell Science, Oxford.

Fry, S. and Johnstone, M.J. (2002) *Ethics in Nursing Practice: A guide to ethical decision making*. Blackwell Science, Oxford.

Giddens, A. (1992) *The Transformation of Intimacy*. Polity Press, Cambridge.

Hendrick, J. (2000) *Law and Ethics in Nursing and Health Care*. Stanley Thornes, Cheltenham.

Hope, T., Savulescu, J. and Hendrick, J. (2003) *Medical Ethics and Law: The core curriculum*. Churchill Livingstone, Edinburgh.

McHale, J. (2001) Consent to treatment 1: General principles. In: *Law and Nursing* (eds J. McHale and J. Tingle). Butterworth-Heinemann, Oxford.

Mason, J.K., McCall Smith, R.A. and Laurie, G.T. (2002) *Law and Medical Ethics*, 6th edn. Butterworths, London.

NMC (2002) *Code of Professional Conduct*. Nursing and Midwifery Council, London.

Parker, M. and Dickenson, D. (2001) *The Cambridge Medical Ethics Workbook*. Cambridge University Press, Cambridge.

Rumbold, G. (1999) *Ethics in Nursing Practice*, 3rd edn. Baillière Tindall, London.

Stauch, M., Wheat, K. and Tingle, J. (2002) *Sourcebook on Medical Law*, 2nd edn. Cavendish, London.

Tschudin V. (2003) *Ethics in Nursing: The caring relationship,* 3rd edn. Butterworth Heinemann, Edinburgh.

Confidentiality and access to medical records

Learning outcomes

By the end of this chapter you should be able to:

- Discuss the duty of confidentiality
- Understand the relationship between confidentiality, privacy and fidelity
- Consider why confidentiality is important
- Identify the situations when confidentiality can be breached

Introduction

To say that confidentiality has long been the cornerstone of good health care is perhaps to state the obvious. Yet even though the principle of confidentiality is widely accepted as one of the most fundamental ethical obligations owed by health professionals it is now more under threat that ever before. In examining why confidentiality is under threat, this chapter discusses what model of confidentiality is appropriate for the 21st century. It also examines why confidentiality is such an important principle. Nevertheless, occasionally other moral and legal considerations may justify breaching (i.e. breaking) confidentiality. What sorts of considerations and what circumstances might be strong enough to override the duty of confidentiality are therefore also discussed. The chapter ends with a brief discussion of patients' rights in respect of their medical records. But, as with other chapters, we start some with some introductory issues, in particular what we mean by the word 'confidential' and how the term is defined in law.

Definitions

~rds

Confidentiality

The principle of keeping secure and secret from others, information given by or about an individual in the course of a professional relationship

What is confidentiality?

As was noted in the introduction, **confidentiality** is one of the most important and well established moral obligations of health-care ethics. According to Gillon (1985), two conditions are necessary to create the moral duty of confidentiality. First, one person must undertake, either expressly or by implication, not to disclose another's secrets (in the sense of information they do not wish to have disclosed without their permission) and second, that other person must disclose to the first person information that s/he considers to be secret.

But what information should you keep secret? Clearly not all information revealed to you is confidential. At least, not that which can be described as part of normal social intercourse (i.e. 'social chit-chat'), or the things that are widely known about people – their marital status, how many children they have and so on (Rumbold 1999). In contrast, personal details about the physical or mental health of your patients (from which they might be identified) is certainly confidential – for example, any symptoms they may be suffering.

Key points **Top tips**

- Realise that confidentiality is a two-way process: this means that some information given to patients is also confidential – i.e. their diagnosis, treatment, nursing care and prognosis
- Remember that confidential information comes in a variety of forms, e.g. in health records (both computer and manual files), medical illustrations, management registers, videos or even in your memory

---

How is confidentiality legally defined?

English courts will generally recognise a legal duty of confidentiality if the following conditions are satisfied (Mason *et al.* 2002). Briefly these are:

- That the information is of a private or intimate nature
- That the information must have been given in a situation where there is an obligation not to disclose it, i.e. it is a fiduciary (trusting) relationship
- There must be an unauthorised use of the information
- That either protecting confidentiality is in the public interest or the patient would suffer if the information was revealed.

According to case law (e.g. *Venables* v. *NGN* [2001]), these conditions mean that the content of records relating to medical, psychological or therapeutic care is, in principle, confidential, including art therapy and group therapy (Montgomery 2003, p. 257).

What are legal sources of confidentiality?

The legal duty of confidentiality arises from several sources:

- The duty of care in negligence (Chapter 5)
- Professional obligations (contained in codes of professional conduct)

- Duties created by various statutes (particularly the Data Protection Act 1998 and the Human Rights Act 1998, see box below)
- Duties in contracts of employment (Dimond 2002).

Data Protection Act 1998 and Human Rights Act 1998

Data Protection Act 1998

The Act provides a framework governing the 'processing' of information that identifies living individuals – 'personal data' in data protection terms. 'Processing' includes holding, obtaining, recording, using and disclosing of information and the Act applies to all forms of media, including paper and images. It applies to confidential patient information but is far wider in its scope, e.g. it also covers personnel records.

The Data Protection Act 1998 imposes constraints on the processing of personal information in relation to living individuals. It identifies eight principles that set out standards for information handling. In the context of confidentiality, the most important principles are:

- The first, which requires processing to be fair and lawful
- The second, which requires personal data to be processed for one or more specified and lawful purposes
- The seventh, which requires personal data to be protected against unauthorised or unlawful processing and against accidental loss, destruction or damage.

Human Rights Act 1998

Article 8 of the Act establishes a right to 'respect for private and family life, home and correspondence'. This underscores the duty to protect the privacy of individuals and preserve the confidentiality of their records. Current understanding is that compliance with the Data Protection Act 1998 and the common law of confidentiality should satisfy human rights requirements.

Legislation generally must also be compatible with the Human Rights Act 1998. This means that any proposal for setting aside obligations of confidentiality must:

- Pursue a legitimate aim
- Be considered necessary in a democratic society
- Be proportionate to the need.

What is whistleblowing?

Whistleblowing occurs when an employee refuses to cover up potentially negligent or harmful practices by drawing attention to them (whether through the media or otherwise). In theory, whistleblowing could be considered a breach of the duty of confidentiality – arising from the employee's contract of employment. Yet, as Tschudin points out (2003, p. 178) it can also result from a health professional taking his/her advocacy role seriously – for which s/he should be rewarded. As Tschudin explains: *'blowing the whistle on unacceptable practice is a professional duty. Is it then not also a professional duty to follow up such acts in a supportive way?'*

Key points Top tips

- The moral duty of confidentiality means that secret or private information must not be disclosed
- The courts will recognise a legal duty of confidentiality if:
    - Information is private
    - There is a fiduciary relationship and
    - The patient will suffer if the information is revealed

Threats to confidentiality

Although there is a long-standing tradition of confidentiality among health professionals that goes back many centuries, the model of confidentiality on which this tradition rests reflects a much simpler pattern of health care than now exists. Thus in the past patients were likely to be treated – possibly for life – by one family doctor and a single specialist at hospital. But now, as group practices replace the single family doctor and treatment in hospital is likely to be delivered by a large number of people, health care is almost always going to involve health professionals working in multidisciplinary teams (McHale 2001). Private hospitals and the voluntary sector are also more likely than in the past to provide services to NHS patients. Developments such as NHS Walk-in Centres and NHS Direct have similarly added to the increasingly flexible pattern of modern medicine. The expanding use of information technology has also contributed to the increasing flow of information.

Given these fundamental changes in health-care delivery it is perhaps not surprising that by the late 1990s there was widespread belief that a more modern approach to protecting patients' confidentiality was required.

⚬━ᴛ Keywords

Caldicott Guardians
Senior health professionals responsible for overseeing the protection of confidentiality in their organisations

New model of confidentiality for the 21st century

The first step towards this new approach was the establishment of a network of so-called **Caldicott Guardians** throughout the NHS.

Given their wide responsibilities and powers (Department of Health 1999), their appointment has been accurately described as a very important, if not essential, step towards recognising the institutional responsibility of the NHS to safeguard confidentiality (Montgomery 2003, p. 253). Following on from this initiative the NHS committed itself to a major programme of investment in a new system for managing confidentiality in the electronic information age. One of the most significant documents to emerge from this process was a new confidentiality code of practice issued in 2003 (see box below).

Confidentiality Code of Practice for NHS Staff (Department of Health 2003)

The code:

- Introduces the concept of confidentiality
- Describes what a confidential service looks like
- Provides a description of the main legal requirements
- Recommends a generic decision support tool for sharing/disclosing information
- Lists examples of particular information sharing experiences.

Key requirements

- **Protect patient information**. Patients' health information and their interests must be protected through a number of measures such as recording information accurately and consistently and keeping patient information private and physically secure.
- **Inform**. Patients must be aware that the information they give may be recorded, may be shared in order to provide them with care, and may be used to support clinical audit and other work to monitor the quality of care provided.
- **Provide choice**. Patients have different needs and values and this must be reflected in the way they are treated both in terms of their medical condition and the handling of personal information.
- **Improve practice**. Because it is not possible to achieve best practice overnight, staff must be aware of the issues surrounding confidentiality and seek training or support where uncertain; they must also report breaches or risk of breaches.

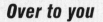

Over to you

Find out who the Caldicott Guardian is in your organisation.

Why is confidentiality important?

In this section we consider why confidentiality is such an important ethical and legal principle.

Consequences for the future

The most common reason given for the moral and legal duty of confidentiality is consequentialist. As such it focuses on the future consequences (to patients and society) if confidentiality is not maintained. Briefly, the claim is that if patients cannot trust you to keep their secrets they will feel betrayed. They are then much more likely to withhold potentially significant but embarrassing details or, worse still, may not seek essential medical or psychiatric care at all (this is especially true in situations where there is a stigma attached to the information disclosed). As a consequence, the care they receive (if any) may not be the most appropriate, not least because, without full and frank disclosure of symptoms and so forth, accurate diagnosis may not be possible. Nor may recommended treatment be the best available if patients have failed to be honest.

Alternatively, patients might reveal very sensitive information but then be very anxious and unhappy that you could reveal it to other people at any time.

As to the effect on society as a whole, the claim is that if a specific patient complains that his/her confidentiality was not maintained – and this becomes widely known – others may lose trust in health professionals. Ultimately this lack of trust could lead to poorer health care for a larger number of people (Hope *et al.* 2003, p. 83).

Respect for patient autonomy

As we saw in Chapter 6, respect for patient autonomy emphasises the right of individuals to decide how their lives are to develop, i.e. according to their own plans, ambitions and so on. In the context of confidentiality, autonomy has to do with how individuals run their lives by controlling what happens to information about themselves – much of which may involve the most intimate aspects of their lives. In other words, they must be entitled to decide what private information should be disclosed (and what should be kept secret).

As Brody says (1997, p. 90), the ability to control information is important because it is bound up with how we relate to other human beings. Or to put it another way, we define and control our relationships by choosing what information to reveal to various people. To some we will reveal very little but to others we may disclose a great deal more (although still not everything).

Privacy

Keywords

Privacy
Respecting privacy means that we should not invade or intrude upon an individual's 'personal space' and should be reluctant to pry

Another reason for the importance of confidentiality is that maintaining confidentiality is a way of protecting a person's **privacy**. Privacy, or rather the right to 'a private life', is a fundamental human right that is now protected by the Human Rights Act 1998 (Article 8). Privacy (like confidentiality) basically allows us to maintain our dignity and integrity by controlling access to ourselves, i.e. choosing what others get to know about us, especially intimate personal details (Beauchamp and Childress 2001).

But privacy is a difficult concept to define precisely. Perhaps the easiest way to understand it is to think of it as a collection of different spaces. The most intimate space (which only the person him/herself has access to) contains the person's most secret thoughts, feelings, hopes fears, etc. Other wider, less private 'spaces'

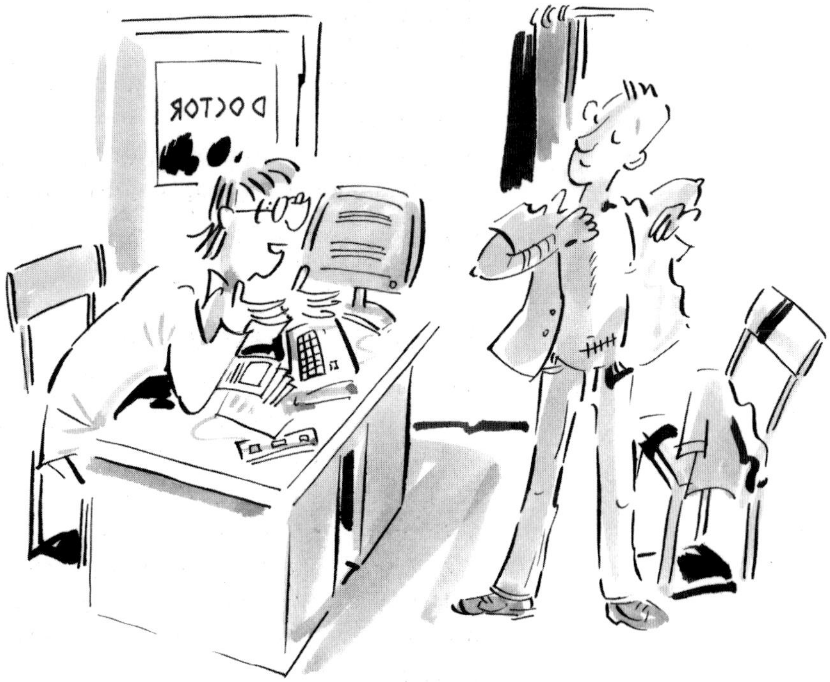

Confidentiality while maintaining privacy.

hold information to which a person's family, friends and so forth have access. And the widest space of all is the public domain, i.e. the space to which the whole world has access (Brown *et al.* 1992, pp. 96–97).

○━π *Keywords*

Fidelity
The ethical principle of fidelity impose obligations that are essential in a trusting relationship, such as keeping promises

Fidelity – a trusting relationship

The final reason for the importance of confidentiality is based on the principle of **fidelity**. One of the most moral important obligations imposed by the principle of fidelity is the obligation to keep your promises (Edwards 1996). This obligation arises because of the nature of the special relationship you have with patients. It is commonly described as a trusting or fiduciary relationship. One of its most basic elements is the promise (albeit often an unspoken, i.e. implied rather than expressed, one) that you will treat information confidentially. Relying on this promise, patients can feel confident that any information they give you will only be revealed with their consent and then only to those with a legitimate interest in it.

Reflective activity

Which 'reason' for confidentiality do you find most convincing? Why? Why do you think it is important to keep promises?

When can confidentiality be breached?

Because there are such good reasons for the duty of confidentiality, you might think that it is an absolute principle, in other words that in no circumstances can it be broken. But this is not the case. In fact every code of professional conduct (as well as the law) recognises situations when you can (and sometimes must) reveal confidential information (Mason *et al.* 2002, p. 243). We will look at two sets of exceptions – those recognised by professional codes and the legal exceptions. As you will see, the two do overlap considerably. Note, too, that the term 'professional' is used in the broadest sense. In this way it can be said to reflect moral considerations.

Professional exceptions – what your code of conduct says about breaching confidentiality

Professional codes of conduct provide very useful guidance about when confidentiality can be broken, for several reasons:

- There are very few legal cases on confidentiality
- Professional codes are often much more precise than the law
- Many problems relating to confidentiality are dealt with more quickly by the professions than by the courts
- Judges have used professional codes in interpreting the law.

The exceptions generally permitted in codes of conduct fall into three categories:

Consent

If patients consent to information being disclosed you can act on that permission, providing it has been freely given. Consent is the most straightforward exception. It is also the most obvious since, as Dimond points out (2002, p. 150), if the duty of confidentiality is owed to the patient it must be in the patient's power to agree to information being disclosed. But if patients refuse to allow disclosure – whether to relatives, the press or employers – you must respect their refusal. Furthermore you should not inform relatives about a patient's diagnosis without first getting the patient's permission (unless, of course, another exception applies).

'Need to know'/patient's interests

Whether described as 'the need to know' or 'patient's interests' this exception to the duty of confidentiality applies when information needs to be shared between all health professionals (and other people, such as social work practitioners) who are involved in a patient's care and treatment. Given the multidisciplinary nature of modern health care the need for this exception is self-evident. But when relying on this exception you must make sure that only those who genuinely 'need to know' – rather than those who are simply curious – are given information. You also need to remember that patients should be told that information about them might have to be shared.

Public interest

O⚊ᴛ *Keywords*

Public interest

The interests of an individual or group of individuals, or of society as a whole, covers, for example, matters such as serious crime or other activities that would put individuals at serious risk of harm

You can disclose confidential information providing it is 'in the **public interest**' to do so.

In practice the public interest exception is the most troublesome. This is because there is no universal definition of what the phrase means. Most commentators agree, however, that very broadly public interest covers matters thought to be 'for the good of society'. Normally this means protecting the public from serious crime and other activities that would put individuals or society at serious risk of harm. Examples typically given in professional guidance as to what amounts to public interest are listed in the first box below. Compare these with those listed in the second box.

Examples of when you can breach confidentiality

To prevent, detect or prosecute:

- Serious crime – murder, manslaughter, kidnapping, child abuse, some sexual and firearm crimes, drug trafficking and so forth
- A threat to national security – serious harm to the security of the state or to public order, including crimes involving substantial financial gain or loss
- Risk of harm – e.g. child abuse or neglect, assault, the spread of infectious diseases, serious fraud or theft involving NHS resources and driving against medical advice
- Disclosures required by law (see below).

Examples of when you should not breach confidentiality

- Casual breaches, e.g. for amusement or through carelessness
- Simply to satisfy another person's curiosity
- To prevent minor crime, or to help conviction in the case of minor crime – most crime against property would probably count as minor crime in this context
- To prevent minor harm to someone else.

Key points **Top tips**

When thinking about breaching patient confidentiality consider:

- Whether it is possible to discuss the issue of disclosure with the individual
- Whether the patient's consent to disclosure could be obtained
- What the likelihood is of harm occurring
- What would be the magnitude of the harm, i.e. how great it is likely to be
- Whether there any other ways (other than breaching confidentiality) of preventing or minimising the harm
- Whether you have followed procedures in your professional code of conduct.

To make sure you respect patient confidentiality remember:

- Not to gossip
- To take care when discussing cases in public places such as on the bus or in a lift
- Not to leave notes open on a desk to be read by all and sundry
- Only to give minimal details on the phone unless you are quite sure of the identity of the caller
- To be very careful when speaking to the press.

- Confidentiality is not an absolute moral principle
- All codes of professional conduct recognise situations when it is ethical to breach patient confidentiality

Legal exceptions

In this section we outline the main legal exceptions to the duty of confidentiality.

Consent

This exception mirrors the professional exception (see above).

Need to know

This exception similarly mirrors the professional exception (see above).

Public interest

The scope of the legal public interest exception – which gives you the option of breaching confidentiality but does not oblige you to – is as uncertain as the professional exception. In other words, there is no single and authoritative legal definition of the phrase 'public interest'. However, the case of *W* v. *Edgell* (1990) provides some general guidelines (see box below).

W v. *Edgell* (1990)

Facts

W was a psychiatric patient who was being detained indefinitely in a secure hospital following his conviction for killing five people 10 years previously. He applied to be discharged and a report on his mental health was prepared by Dr Edgell. Dr Edgell strongly opposed W's transfer to a regional secure unit – the first step towards his eventual release – because of his long-standing and continuing abnormal interest in firearms and home-made bombs. In short, Edgell claimed that W was still a very dangerous man. In fact he was so concerned that, even though W withdrew his application, Edgell sent a copy of the report to the medical director of the hospital and the Home Office. W sued Edgell for breach of confidentiality.

Court's decision

W lost his action. The court held that the duty of confidentiality owed to W was outweighed by the overriding interest in public safety. The court would, of course, have decided differently if Edgell had, without concealing W's identity, sold 'his story' to the newspapers.

continued

The guidelines established by *W* v. *Edgell* about the scope of 'public interest' in law can be summarised as follows:

- Before disclosure can be justified there must be a 'real', immediate and serious risk of danger to the public
- Disclosure must be limited to those with a legitimate interest in receiving the information
- Only such confidential information as is strictly necessary should be revealed, not more
- Arguably, the risk to the public must be to their physical safety, i.e. danger of physical harm or disease.

The *Edgell* case was controversial but has been followed – see, for example, *R* v. *Crozier* (1990); *X* v. *Y* (1988); *Woolgar* v. *Chief Constable of Sussex Police* (1999).

Disclosures to the police

There is no general legal duty to report crime to the police. This means that that you do not have to volunteer information to them if, say, a patient tells you that he has committed a crime. Nevertheless, you must not obstruct police investigations (e.g. give false or misleading information). Note that refusing to answer their questions with a 'lawful' excuse is not obstruction – the lawful excuse being your duty of confidentiality.

Relevant here too is the Police and Criminal Evidence Act 1984, under which medical records (and diagnostic samples) are subject to special procedures. These are designed to protect patient confidentiality and mean that, if the police want to see such records, they have to get permission from a judge.

Statutory obligations

Several statutes impose obligations on health professionals to breach confidentiality. These include legislation to:

- Combat terrorism
- Identify drivers who have committed traffic offences (Road Traffic Act 1988)
- Notify authorities of births and deaths (Births and Deaths Registration Act 1953)
- Report 'notifiable diseases', e.g. cholera, plague, food poisoning (Public Health (Control of Disease) Act 1984)
- Provide information about abortions (Abortion Act 1967).

Other statutory provisions governing disclosure include the Children Act 1989 and the Human Fertilisation and Embryology Act 1990. Note also that the Health Act 1999 and the Health and Social Care

Act 2001contain provisions for breaching confidentiality (for further details of these and other statutory provisions see Montgomery 2003, pp. 273–276).

Civil proceedings and court orders

Sometimes health records may be relevant in civil proceedings, particularly in negligence claims and child protection cases. Unless these are volunteered, a court order may be issued. You then have no option but to disclose the relevant information. Note that you may also be required to give evidence in court – even though that evidence involves revealing confidential information – as happened in *Re C.* (1991). The case concerned the proposed adoption of a 1-year-old baby. A day before the adoption hearing the mother withdrew her consent to the adoption. The adopting parents' solicitor then produced a document, sworn voluntarily by the mother's GP, containing evidence of her mental condition and fitness to bring up a child. The mother objected to this evidence being admitted, claiming it was a breach of her medical confidentiality. She lost her action as the court held that the GP's evidence was highly relevant. In short, the child's welfare – and the need for the court to have all relevant information – outweighed the duty of confidentiality owed to the mother.

Reflective activity

Consider whether you would breach confidentiality in the following situations. Give reasons for your decisions.

- A colleague has confided in you that she has 'a drink problem'
- Working in the community you discover a patient has received stolen goods worth about £10 000
- One of your patients, a 3-year-old girl, has a broken wrist and several bruises. You think (but are not sure) that these may have been caused by her stepfather
- Recently diagnosed with an inherited disorder – which is very serious but treatable – a patient refuses to give her consent to you revealing this information to her husband.

Key points   *Top tips*

- Confidentiality is not an absolute legal principle, i.e. there may be circumstances when you can reveal confidential information

What patients can do when their confidentiality is breached

Few patients have ever taken legal action to enforce their rights to confidentiality. In principle, legal remedies are available – both to stop a threatened breach and where a breach has already occurred. Threatened breaches can be stopped by an injunction. An injunction – the so-called 'gagging order' – is an order that requires someone either to do or to stop doing a particular act. An alternative remedy is damages – which might only be minimal unless the patient can show loss of society, severe injury to feelings, job loss, interference with prospects of promotion or the like (Mason *et al.* 2002, p. 265). Usually, however, the most effective remedy is for patients to lodge a complaint alleging professional misconduct, which could result in disciplinary proceedings and possibly dismissal.

Medical records

The relationship of trust and confidence that you have with your patients is a two-way process. One element is the duty of confidentiality. The other, which is equally important if patients are to have control over their health care, is the right to know what information has been complied about them.

In the past there was considerable opposition to patients having access to their records. It was asserted, for example, that patients would not understand medical records; they would be frightened (by technical language, medical shorthand or poor prognosis); or that health professionals would not be able to make 'frank' comments. But by the early 1980s attitudes had changed and the Data Protection Act 1984 was passed. The Act gave patients the right to see their medical records and was the first of several statutes recognising the principle of patient access.

There are several reasons why patients now regard access to their medical records as a fundamental right. First, much more information is routinely collected and stored than ever before. As a result more confidential information – some of which may be very sensitive (and thus potentially harmful if it got into the 'wrong' hands) – is widely accessible. Second, information stored on record is sometimes inaccurate or misleading. Not surprisingly therefore patients expect to 'set the record straight' or at least check on what has been said about them, especially if they suspect that a defamatory remark has been made about them.

Although patients do not have any general rights under the common law to see their health records, several statutes do grant such rights. Of these the most important are:

- The Data Protection Act 1998
- The Access to Health Records Act 1990
- The Access to Medical Reports Act 1988.

Data Protection Act 1998

This Act (which replaces the 1984 Act) gives every living person the right to apply for access to their health records. A health record (which includes both NHS and private health sector records) is defined as a record consisting of information about the physical or mental health or condition of an identifiable individual made by or on behalf of a health professional in connection with the care of that individual. You should note that the Act refers to personal data (a term that includes health records but is much broader). Not surprisingly, the term 'health professional' is defined very broadly too. It includes doctors, nurses, dentists, midwives, health visitors, occupational therapists, physiotherapists, art and music therapists and so on.

The Act allows patients to be:

- Informed whether personal data is processed
- Given a description of the data held, the purposes for which it is processed and to whom the data may be disclosed
- Given a copy of the information constituting the data
- Given information on the source of the data.

The Act also contains detailed provisions about the procedure to be followed to gain access to health records (including time limits, cost, etc.). But the important point to note is that information contained in a record can be withheld in certain circumstances. In particular, access can be denied (or limited) where the information might cause serious harm to the physical or mental health or condition of the 'data subject' or any other person.

Over to you

Go to the Department of Health website at www.doh.gov.uk/confiden/ and answer the following questions:

- Describe the various ways health records can be recorded
- When information has been withheld, what do patients have to be told?
- Can patients directly inspect their records?
- Do patients have to explain why they want access to their records?
- What can patients do if they feel their medical records are incorrect?

Access to Health Records Act 1990

Largely replaced by the Data Protection Act 1998, the only relevance now of the 1990 Act is to the records of deceased persons (for a discussion of confidentiality and death see Mason *et al.* 2002, pp. 267–70).

Access to Medical Reports Act 1988

This Act applies to reports prepared by doctors for employment or insurance purposes. It says that such reports can only be supplied with the patient's knowledge and consent. In other words, patients have the right to see the report, subject to certain safeguards, before it is supplied and can then ask for it to be altered (for further details see Montgomery 2003, pp. 284–286).

Key points Top tips

- Several statutes give patients a legal right to see their health records
- Patients' legal rights to see their health records is not absolute, i.e. access may be denied in certain circumstances

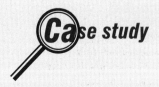
Case study

Must you respect Tony's confidentiality?

Tony, one of your patients, is HIV-positive. Devastated by the news, he refuses to consent to his partner, Carol, being told even though he knows she may become infected. You know that great efforts have been made to persuade Tony to tell Carol but he still refuses to change his mind. However, you think that Carol has the right to know.

Reflective activity

1. Must Tony's demand for privacy be respected or can you justify breaching his confidentiality by telling Carol of his HIV status?
2. Would it make any difference if Tony was not HIV-positive but had a sexually transmitted disease instead?

Case study continued

1. Telling Carol

Your moral responsibility

Several different approaches could be taken. You could decide that the duty of confidentiality is an absolute moral principle that should not be breached for any reason. Another approach is to treat it as a qualified principle, which would mean that confidentiality could be breached in certain circumstances (e.g. if someone would otherwise be seriously harmed). Alternatively (an approach that falls somewhere between the two) you could do all you can to protect Carol while at the same time maintaining Tony's confidentiality. You could, for example, try to persuade Tony to take appropriate precautions and not take risks such as having 'unsafe sex'.

But if after careful reflection you decide to tell Carol of Tony's HIV status you will have to justify your decision. The exception to the duty of confidentiality that you would normally rely in this kind of case would be the 'public interest' one, i.e. breaching confidentiality is necessary to protect Carol from serious risk of harm. In justifying your decision you would, of course, have to consider that the risk of transmission depends on various factors.

Your legal responsibility

Your legal responsibility would also depend on the 'public interest' exception. There has been no case directly on this issue. Nonetheless, despite the uncertainty as to the legal scope of the term 'public interest', most legal commentators (e.g. Mason *et al.* 2002, Dimond 2002) assert that passing on information to a patient's partner – even without consent – is allowable so long as every effort has been made to persuade the patient to do so and there is a 'real and serious' risk to a specific person.

2. Tony's sexually transmitted disease

Your moral and legal responsibility would again turn on whether – relying on the 'public interest' exception – there is a good enough reason to breach your duty of confidentiality to Tony. In reaching your decision you would have to bear in mind that it would be harder to justify doing so if Tony was suffering from a disease that, although infectious, was not fatal. Nevertheless, relevant here would be such factors as, for example, how great was the risk of transmission and what impact the disease could have on Carol's fertility.

Reflective activity

Why is it appropriate to describe the choice you need to make about breaching Tony's confidentiality as a dilemma (see Chapter 1 for the definition of a dilemma)?

The case study implies that Carol was not one of your patients. What difference would it make if she were?

The relationship between law and ethics

Similarities between law and ethics

- **Justification**. The ethical and legal duty of confidentiality can be justified on both consequentialist and deontological grounds (i.e. on the basis of respect for autonomy and privacy).

- **Breaching confidentiality**. In neither law nor ethics is confidentiality regarded as an absolute principle; rather it is qualified. That means there may be good reasons to break a patient's confidentiality.

- **Exceptions to duty of confidentiality**. The legal and ethical grounds for breaching confidentiality are broadly similar and include:

  - Consent

  - 'Need to know'

  - 'Public interest'

  - Disclosures required by statute or court order.

Differences between law and ethics

- **Origins**. The moral duty to protect patient confidentiality goes back to the 5th century BC. The legal sources of confidentiality are much more recent.

- **Sanctions**. Professional sanctions, e.g. disciplinary proceedings, are much quicker and more effective than legal remedies.

- **Clarity**. Professional codes and guidelines about the scope, nature and exceptions to the duty of confidentiality are usually much clearer than the law.

Rapid recap

Check your progress so far by working through each of the following questions.

1. What is confidentiality?
2. Why is confidentiality important?
3. What is the purpose of the 2003 NHS confidentiality code of practice?
4. Is confidentiality an absolute principle?
5. What is meant by the 'public interest'?

If you have difficulty with more than one of the questions, read through the section again to refresh your understanding before moving on.

References

Beauchamp, T.L. and Childress, J.F. (2001) *Principles of Biomedical Ethics*, 5th edn. Oxford University Press, Oxford.

Brody, H. (1997) The physician–patient relationship. In: *Medical Ethics* (ed. R. Veatch). Jones & Bartlett, Sudbury.

Brown, J.M., Kitson, A.L. and McKnight, T.J. (1992) *Challenges in Caring*. Chapman & Hall, London.

Department of Health (1999) *HSC 99/012*. HMSO, London.

Department of Health (2003) *National Health Service Confidentiality Code of Practice*. HMSO, London.

Dimond, B. (2002) *Legal Aspects of Midwifery*, 2nd edn. Books for Midwives, Edinburgh.

Edwards, S.D. (1996) *Nursing Ethics: A principle-based approach*. Macmillan, Basingstoke.

Gillon, R. (1985) *Philosophical Medical Ethics*. John Wiley, Chichester.

Hope, T., Savulescu, J. and Hendrick, J. (2003) *Medical Ethics and Law: The core curriculum*. Churchill Livingstone, Edinburgh.

McHale, J. (2001) Confidentiality and access to health records. In: *Law and Nursing* (eds J. McHale and J. Tingle). Butterworth-Heinemann, Oxford.

Mason, J.K., McCall Smith, R.A. and Laurie, G.T. (2002) *Law and Medical Ethics*, 6th edn. Butterworths, London.

Montgomery, J. (2003) *Health Care Law*. Oxford University Press, Oxford.

Rumbold, G. (1999) *Ethics in Nursing Practice*, 3rd edn. Baillière Tindall, London.

Tschudin V. (2003) *Ethics in Nursing: The caring relationship*, 3rd edn. Butterworth Heinemann, Edinburgh.

8

Clinical research

Introduction

There can be few people who are unaware of the so-called 'mercy deaths', including 'euthanasia by starvation' and gassing of those considered 'racially impure' in mental hospitals in Germany during the 1930s and 1940s. The full horrors of the appalling experiments carried out by Nazi doctors on concentration camp inmates during the Second World War (and in Japan during the same period) are also now well known. These caused immense pain and suffering, disability and often death but provided very little useful scientific knowledge. But how could scientists and doctors have carried out such atrocities? The underlying reason behind such actions seems to have been the belief that certain groups of people were worthless, had no individual value and so could be sacrificed for some 'common good' such as the advancement of medicine (Campbell *et al.* 2001).

It is to avoid such actions ever happening again that the most famous and earliest international code on the ethics of research, the Nuremberg Code, was drawn up in 1949. As this chapter will explain, this code (and subsequent international and national guidelines) is just one of several safeguards designed to prevent abuse in research. Others include the NHS research governance framework and research ethics committees. The role of the law in regulating research will similarly be explained but the chapter begins with some introductory issues – the definition of research and the moral issues it raises. How you may become involved in the research process is also briefly discussed. Note that this chapter does not deal with research involving children under 18 and incompetent adults (these are covered in Chapters 11 and 12).

What is research?

Types of research

Surprisingly perhaps, the term 'research' is not easy to define precisely. This is because it is commonly used interchangeably with a variety of other terms (such as evaluation, clinical audit, experimentation and even quality assurance) to describe processes by which information is collected and analysed. That said, it is broadly agreed that **research** involves systematic enquiry aimed at discovering new facts about the way things in the world around us behave (Stauch *et al.* 2002, p. 549). Because research is thus associated with 'progress, 'discovery' and 'improvement', it is generally seen as a good thing.

Traditionally, two types of research have been recognised: therapeutic and non-therapeutic research.

- **Therapeutic research** aims to benefit patients by, for example, using new methods or a new procedure that is more likely to cure their disease or improve their condition. As such, it combines research with the care and treatment of patients.
- **Non-therapeutic research** aims principally to gain scientific knowledge. Typically it involves testing new drugs. However, whatever form it takes, this type of research is unlikely to benefit the research subjects personally.

Although it is still common to distinguish between therapeutic and non-therapeutic research, the distinction has been challenged in recent years on the grounds that the boundaries between the two are often blurred in practice. However, there are sound arguments for retaining the distinction. First, almost all ethical guidelines and codes covering research do so. Second, the distinction is crucial in weighing the risks and benefits of a particular project. Third, the nature of the project can determine the amount of information that should be disclosed (see below).

But whether the research is therapeutic or non-therapeutic it should be distinguished from what is known as innovative treatment. Innovative treatment is much more speculative than research and generally lacks the necessary systematic and repetitive quality to count as proper research (Stauch *et al.* 2002, p. 552).

Another distinction sometimes made is between invasive and non-invasive research. Invasive research is essentially any activity that involves bodily contact. Non-invasive research does not involve any such contact and so includes activities such as conducting surveys, observation, researching into medical records and so on.

⊙━ᴛ *Keywords*

Research
An attempt to obtain new knowledge by addressing clearly defined questions with systematic and rigorous methods

Types of research subject

There are four types of research subject:

- Individual patients
- Groups of patients suffering from a particular condition
- Patients who have no association with the condition under review but who are readily available (so-called patient volunteers)
- Healthy volunteers.

Purpose of research

The purpose of all medical research is:

- To benefit society by understanding the causes of disease or dysfunction
- To find effective methods of prevention and treatment (BMA 2001, p. 205).

Indeed, it is widely acknowledged that without research many of the key advances in the last century would never have happened (Mason *et al.* 2002). That said, it is also important to bear in mind that, although the ultimate goal of medical research must be to find complete cures, the reality is that research is almost always going to take the form of 'steps on the way' to complete cures rather than reaching the goal in one go. As Foster wisely says (2001, p. 1): *'giant leaps in understanding and treatment are not, by their very nature, planned, as the story of penicillin's discovery demonstrates. Meanwhile the pedestrian plodding of routine research has to go on.'*

Your role in research

You can act in a range of roles in research:

- Undertaking research yourself, i.e. conducting your own trials
- Practising in settings where research is being carried out, i.e. caring for patients enrolled in trials
- Taking part in research yourself – as a healthy volunteer
- Acting as a manager or executive – enabling you to, for example, commission research studies or supervise less experienced researchers
- Acting as a member of a research ethics committee.

Each of these roles will carry particular duties and responsibilities. But irrespective of your precise role your primary responsibility is for the research subject (Ashcroft 2002, p. 278). This means that you must practise within an ethical framework. What then are the ethical principles that guide research? Or to put it another way, how can you be sure research is ethical?

How can you be sure research is ethical?

To be ethical research must be based on the following considerations and principles:

Respect for autonomy

As we saw in Chapter 6, respect for autonomy is one of the most fundamental moral principles in health care. Treating individuals with respect means that they must have the right to make their own reasoned decisions according to their own goals and values. In research situations this means that participants must give informed consent, i.e. their participation must be:

- Voluntary and free from coercion
- Fully informed
- Private/confidential.

Voluntary and free from coercion

Consent can only be free and voluntary if researchers do not threaten, trick people into unwittingly participating or offer them excessive rewards. Nor should existing patients be persuaded to take part in research for fear of reprisals if they refuse – that their care and treatment may be compromised or that they will be discriminated against in some way. Note too that participants must be aware that they have the right to withdraw from the study at any time.

Fully informed

To make free and rational choices participants need adequate information. They have the right, in short, to be 'fully informed'. What this means is that potential participants have the right to full and frank replies to the following questions:

- What is the purpose of the study?
- Why they have been chosen?
- What will happen if they take part?
- What do they have to do?
- What is the drug or procedure that is being tested?
- What are the alternatives for diagnosis or treatment?
- What are the side effects of any treatment received when taking part?
- What are the possible disadvantages and risks of taking part?
- What are the possible benefits?

- What happens when the research study stops?
- What if something goes wrong?
- What will happen to the results of the research study?
- Will taking part be kept confidential (see further Department of Health 2001)?

Privacy/confidentiality

Where people are the focus of research, their right to privacy is a critical issue. Attention to privacy means safeguarding participants' dignity by making sure that they decide when, where and what kind of information is shared. In other words, their confidentiality and anonymity must be protected. Note that confidentiality applies to a broad range of data, including written medical records, photographic, videotape and electronic material, human tissue and so on.

It is also important to stress that protecting confidentiality means making sure that information is only used for the purposes of the research study and so should not be made public or available to anyone other than those involved in the research process without the participants' consent (see Chapter 7).

Justice

Justice is about fairness. In research situations the factors you need to consider in ensuring fair treatment are:

- **Selection process**. Participants should be selected on the basis of research needs rather than because they are disadvantaged, i.e. poor or institutionalised and therefore cheaper, easier or simply more convenient to use
- **Distribution of risks and benefits**. The distribution of risks and benefits must be as fair as possible, i.e. no one group should benefit overwhelmingly or be discriminated against – e.g. because of age, gender, race or ethnic background
- **Support**. Participants should be supported both during the research and after it has ended. Accordingly, they should have access to professional support and advice if, for example, they suffer adverse side effects.

Beneficence and non-maleficence – balancing risks and benefits

Briefly the principles of beneficence (to do 'good') and non-maleficence (not to harm) mean that participants' health and well-being must be safeguarded and promoted. Applying these principles in practice basically involves carrying out a balancing exercise. In other words, the risks and benefits have to be compared to make sure that any risk of harm is in proportion to the potential benefits. The key concepts here are, of course, risk of harm and benefit. What do these terms mean in research situations?

Risk of harm

Harm can take many forms – it can be physical, mental, emotional and spiritual. As such it can range from the most devastating physical symptoms to less serious states of mind (such as embarrassment and so forth). All these types of harm can be temporary or involve more permanent injury, disability or discomfort. In some cases the harm can be financial – loss of income, for example. But in others it may be very difficult to assess – such as when it involves loss of privacy or time. But however it is defined there can be little doubt that the principle of non-maleficence (the obligation to do no harm) makes it very difficult, if not impossible, to ever justify using human research subjects. This is because any intervention, however small, risks causing some harm. On the other hand, failing to carry out any research at all clearly goes against the principle of beneficence, in so far as patients and society will be denied the knowledge and understanding gained through research.

Benefit

There may be several benefits of research. First among these is an improvement in the health of patients – their symptoms may be relieved or, better still, their condition may be cured. But sometimes the benefits may only become apparent long after the research has been completed and so are unlikely to lead to any immediate changes in practice. They may nevertheless lead to improved care and treatment in the future. Alternatively, if the research is non-therapeutic, society rather than the individual may benefit.

Given the potential conflict between beneficence and non-maleficence, it is clear, then, that a balancing exercise has to be carried out. So what does this involve?

Balancing risks/benefits

The purpose of balancing risks and benefits is to make sure that participants are only involved in research when the benefits clearly outweigh the possible risks. Yet, if we accept that there is an element of risk in all interventions (although the amount of risk varies greatly according to the nature of the research), what we really need to know is: What is an acceptable level of risk? The answer to this question depends on whether the research is non-therapeutic or therapeutic.

Keywords

Minimal risk
A small chance of a reaction that itself is trivial, or a very remote chance of more serious injury

Professional guidance in relation to non-therapeutic research generally advises that patients should not be subjected to more than '**minimal risk**'.

A risk is minimal if it involves risk of injury or death that is no greater than that faced in everyday life – such as a headache or a feeling of lethargy.

As regards therapeutic research, if the level of risk rises above minimal risk, then patients should be involved only if:

- The risk is still small in comparison with that already incurred by the patient as a consequence of the disease itself
- The disease is a serious one
- The knowledge gained from the research is likely to be of great practical benefit
- There is no other means of obtaining that knowledge; and
- The patient gives fully informed consent (Mason *et al.* 2002, p. 574).

Key points | **Top tips**

- Balancing risks and benefits is a very complex process; for further guidance visit the Medical Research Council website at: www.mrc.ac.uk

Scientific validity

To have scientific validity research must be:

- Well designed
- Based on sound knowledge and proper scientific methods
- Carried out by properly qualified researchers.

As Ashcroft explains (2002, p. 281), a well-designed study is one that is both reliable and likely to answer the research question. However, it may be that a particular study, while well designed, will ultimately serve no useful purpose (because the research question itself is pointless). If so it will almost certainly be unethical. Similarly, a poorly designed project that could produce significant benefits will also be unethical. In this case it is unethical because the lack of proper scientific methods means that it is unlikely to answer the research question (Royal College of Nursing 2003).

Reflective activity

Should journals refuse to publish the results of a study that is unethical because participants were not fully informed of the risks? Justify your answer.

The key ethical principles and considerations in research are:

- Respect for autonomy
- Justice
- Risk/benefit analysis
- Scientific validity.

Regulation of research

Research is 'regulated' in several different ways – by ethical codes, NHS research governance, research ethics committees and the law of consent. As you will see, these various mechanisms supplement each other (and overlap).

Ethical codes and professional guidelines

The Nuremberg Code (1949) – undoubtedly the most famous international code and the first to provide guidance on the ethical principles that should govern research – has been hugely influential. The code was later supplemented by the Declaration of Helsinki, first drawn up in 1964 but revised several times since then (most recently in 2003). But, despite being widely known, neither of these codes have eliminated abuse. Indeed, infamous examples of abusive and harmful research are well documented – with trials of AIDS drugs and vaccines being the latest to cause concern (Campbell *et al.* 2001). The potential for abuse explains perhaps why there are now such a huge range of ethical codes and guidelines regulating research. These include international and national guidelines published by medical and professional bodies as well as the government (in the UK alone there are now at least 40 such sets – British Medical Association 2001).

Not surprisingly, ethical guidelines and codes vary in length, focus and detail. Yet, as Hope *et al.* point out (2003, p. 194), several key principles are consistently emphasised. These are that:

- The research must be scientifically sound
- It must satisfy the proportionality test, i.e. benefits must clearly outweigh possible harms
- No coercion must be brought to bear on potential participants
- Participants must be fully informed
- Payments may be made only to offset reasonable costs (and must not be used to induce people to take part).

Key points **Top tips**

When reading codes and professional guidelines on research, think about how they:

- Define the moral obligations of researchers
- Emphasise the right of participants
- Provide strong evidence of best practice

Key points **Top tips**

- For guidance on worldwide agreements on research ethics visit the World Medical Assembly website at: www.wma.net

National Health Service research governance

National Health Service research governance for health and social care was first introduced in 2001 as one of the main responses to a public scandal involving research on children at North Staffordshire Hospital. Revised in 2004, the governance framework applies to all research, clinical and non-clinical, carried out by NHS staff using NHS resources (as well as that carried out by other groups including industry and universities within health-care systems). Research governance aims to improve research quality and safeguard the public by:

- Enhancing ethical and scientific quality
- Promoting good practice
- Reducing adverse incidents and ensuring that lessons are learned
- Preventing poor performance.

In an important change from previous Department of Health guidance on research, the governance framework is very broad in scope. Consequently, it does not only apply to those who undertake research (or manage and fund it) but also to all health professionals who 'are responsible for the care of participants in the research'. Not surprisingly, the fundamental principles identified in the governance framework 'as the key to ethical research' echo those in ethical codes and professional guidelines. In other words, they emphasise how the dignity, rights, safety and well-being of participants must be the primary consideration in any research study.

Top tips

- You can find out more about the NHS research governance framework on line at: www.dh.gov.uk/

Research ethics committees

Almost all research guidelines recognise the need for some form of independent review to vet the ethical aspects of research. Since 1968 local research ethics committees (LRECs) have performed this task. There is no doubt that these committees have had a positive impact on the conduct of research – especially through their insistence on the provision of full and clear information to participants (Fox 2002). Yet they have also been criticised. In the past most of the criticisms focused on how practices varied too widely. In other words, the committees operated in isolation from each other with little or no coordination (Neuberger 1992). More recent criticism has focused on the process of ethical review itself. According to Foster (2001, p. 141), for example, the more the process of reviewing research proposals has shifted away from individual researchers to a committee, the more moral thinking has become 'lazy'. As Foster explains, this shift (from individual responsibility to collective responsibility) means: *'that the process of ethical review becomes more a process of following rules than a reflective practice . . . once rules are written most people tend not to think about why they take the form they do or whether they are really good rules or not'.*

It is too early to assess the impact of current guidance regulating research ethics committees (called *Governance Arrangements for National Health Service Research Ethics Committees*, Department of Health 2001). Certainly it is very detailed and wide ranging – covering all research involving patients and users of the NHS. The guidance includes sections on membership requirements and composition, working procedures, support and education and how/when to apply for ethical review and so on. In this context, however, the most important aspect of the guidance is the advice it gives RECs about their role in ensuring that research proposals are ethical. These are summarised in the box below.

Governance Arrangements for National Health Service Research Ethics Committees (Department of Health 2001)

Before giving a favourable opinion the research ethics committee should be adequately reassured about the following issues:

- **The scientific design and conduct of the study**. In other words, it must be appropriate, statistically sound, predictable and risks must be weighed against expected benefits.
- **Recruitment**. This covers the characteristics of the population from which participants will be drawn (including age, gender, culture and so on) and the justifications for any decisions made in this respect.
- **Care and protection**. This focuses on, for example, the safety of any intervention, the suitability of the researchers, plans to withhold or withdraw standard therapies, support of participants during and after research is completed, financial considerations.
- **Informed consent**. The requires scrutiny of the process of obtaining consent – the adequacy and understandability of written and oral information, how queries are dealt with and so on.
- **Community considerations**. These include the impact/relevance of the research to local and concerned communities from which the participants are drawn, steps taken to consult these communities, etc.

N.B. New operating procedures for research ethics committees were introduced in March 2004. These were necessary to meet EU Directive 2001/20/EC covering clinical trials of medicinal products.

Top tips

- *Governance Arrangements for National Health Service Research Ethics Committees should be read in conjunction with the NHS research governance framework for health and social care*
- *You can keep up to date about developments relevant to RECs by accessing the Central Office for Research Ethics Committees (Corec) website at: www.corec.org.uk*

Key points

- The main function of a research ethics committee is to advise health bodies on the ethical acceptability of research
- Research ethics committees are responsible for acting primarily in the interests of potential research participants

The legal regulation of research

In this section we discuss the law's role in regulating research. As you will see, this focuses on the law of consent.

The law of consent

There is no specific legislation governing research on humans other than that covering clinical trials (see below). This means that, in addition to the general duty of care (see Chapter 5) owed by health professionals (and the law of confidentiality), the legal regulation of research is in effect the law relating to consent. In other words, participants must rely on common law principles of consent to protect them from unethical research and if research involves any physical contact with participants it will be unlawful unless their consent is obtained beforehand. If no consent at all is obtained, a researcher could face criminal charges and a civil action. More likely, however, is a claim by a participant that, although consent was given, it was flawed in some way. In such cases a negligence action may be possible (see Chapter 5).

In practice, the aspects of consent law that are the most problematic in research situations focus on competency and information disclosure.

Competency – how do you know adult participants are competent?

There seems little doubt that the test for competency that applies in respect of treatment applies equally to research, both therapeutic and non-therapeutic. In other words, in the absence of evidence to the contrary (and until the Mental Capacity Bill 2004 comes into force) adult patients are competent if they are capable of comprehending and retaining information, of believing it and of weighing it up (see *Re C* [1994] and Chapter 6).

Information disclosure – how much information must a researcher reveal?

As yet there has been no case before the English courts on the legal standard of disclosure. It is therefore not possible to say precisely what research participants can expect to be told. But notwithstanding the uncertainty of the law most legal texts assume that, if faced with deciding the appropriate standard of disclosure, the courts would probably choose an 'informed consent' approach, i.e. a 'reasonable' pro-participant standard rather than a professional-led one (Mason *et al.* 2002, Montgomery 2003). Indeed, for the courts to do otherwise would mean going against all current ethical codes and professional guidelines as to what is considered 'accepted or responsible practice'.

In the meantime (until there is legislation or the courts decide the issue), researchers should assume that the law requires a full and frank disclosure of information. This means that, if the research is therapeutic, patients should be given the following information:

- The purpose of the research
- That their care and treatment is being combined with research
- Benefits to participants and society
- Risks involved, in particular those that a 'reasonable' patient volunteering for the risks research would want to know
- Alternatives open to the participants
- Any other significant consequence of the research, e.g. that they may have to stay longer in hospital or return for more frequent check-ups.

Key points | **Top tips**

- Be aware that the more severe the patient's illness the greater the risks that can lawfully be taken
- It will normally be up to patients themselves to determine the risk:benefit ratio (Kennedy and Grubb 2000, p. 1717)

As regards non-therapeutic research, full and frank disclosure means that researchers must not only provide all the information they would normally provide participants in therapeutic research but also give details of all the risks that the actual participants want to know about. In other words, the law requires a more subjective approach than is required for therapeutic research.

Clinical trials

Clinical trials are now governed by the Medicines for Human Use (Clinical Trials) Regulations 2004. The definition of a 'clinical trial' is very technical but basically the focus of the regulations is the type of research required to justify the licensing of medicinal products (Montgomery 2003, p. 358). A simpler explanation of a clinical trial is Kennedy and Grubb's (2000, p. 1708) – it is when:

- A doctor tests the efficacy of a new treatment where none has previously been available and the patient would otherwise have received ordinary nursing care and symptomatic relief but nothing else

- A doctor tests the efficacy of a new treatment as against other established forms of treatment; or
- A doctor tests treatments A, B and C (all of which are established) because it has not been established which is the most efficacious.

However, as Montgomery points out (2003, p. 358), because in practice it is difficult to distinguish the procedure for approving clinical trials from other forms of research, it is likely that the new legal framework will be used for all health-care research.

The regulations identify two main safeguards to protect participants from unethical research. These are informed consent and ethics committee approval (see further Parts 2 and 3, and Schedule 1 of the Medicines for Human Use (Clinical Trials) Regulations 2004).

Key points | Top tips

- Research is only lawful if participants' consent is first obtained
- Research is governed by common law principles of consent
- Clinical trials are regulated by the Medicines for Human Use (Clinical Trials) Regulations 2004

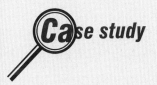

Case study

Michael and the randomised controlled trial

Michael has a degenerative neurological disorder and has recently found it increasingly difficult to walk. Existing treatment is having little impact on his mobility and a randomised controlled trial (RCT) has been set up. Michael is very keen to be involved – so keen that he barely listens to the information he is given during a short talk about the new drug (which focuses only on its potential benefits). Michael does, however, make it clear that he wants to try the new drug in the hope that it might make it easier for him to walk.

You are part of a multidisciplinary team caring for Michael but are worried that the RCT (which is double-blind) has not been properly explained to him. In fact, you know that Michael is under the impression that he will definitely get the new drug.

Reflective activity

1. What is an RCT?
2. What ethical issues does an RCT raise?
3. When is an RCT lawful?

Case study continued

1. Definition of a randomised controlled trial

In an RCT patients are allocated into groups at random. One group (the experimental or treatment group) gets the new drug and another group (the control group) will be given the standard treatment, a placebo (pretend medicine) or no treatment at all. The fundamental purpose of an RCT is to make comparisons between the groups. In double-blind trials neither the researcher nor the participant knows which drug the participant has been given until the trial is over.

2. Ethical issues

Even the best-designed RCT has a built-in moral dilemma – whether it is ever justifiable to deny the control group the potential benefit of the new treatment. In other words, is it ethical to deprive Michael (who, given the random nature of the trial, may only be getting the standard treatment, a placebo or no treatment at all)? Similarly, is it ethical to give a relatively untried new drug (which may harm them) to the treatment group, while on the other hand denying them existing treatment, which may be of some, albeit limited, benefit? Given these moral dilemmas it is clear that no randomised therapeutic trial can be ethical unless health professionals genuinely cannot agree which treatment yields the best results (Mason *et al.* 2002, p. 580). It is essential, too, that the trial is stopped as soon as an adverse effect becomes clear.

The other major ethical concern in this case study focuses on consent. It seems unlikely that Michael understands the nature of an RCT or indeed any of the other issues that are normally discussed in patient information sheets (see e.g. Department of Health 2001). Does he, for example, know about the risks associated with the new drug?

Taking into account all these factors – and the requirements of the *Research Governance Framework for Health and Social Care* (Department of Health 2004) on the consent process – it is very unlikely that it is ethical to enter Michael into the RCT.

3. The legality of a randomised controlled trial

As Kennedy and Grubb (2000, p. 1708) point out, because clinical trials involve a doctor–patient relationship, the duty of the doctor to act in the best interests of his/her patient applies. This has certain consequences:

● If the trial consists of testing a new treatment, the doctor must have reasonable grounds for believing that the new treatment may be efficacious

● Patients not receiving any new treatment (i.e. those in the control group) must receive the best available established treatment

● The trial must contain an appropriate mechanism whereby it can be discontinued if a) a new treatment proves less beneficial than the established treatment or b) a new treatment proves more beneficial than existing therapies or the best available other.

A further legal concern raised by the RCT focuses on whether Michael can be given enough information to satisfy the legal standard of disclosure. For consent to be legally valid in relation to therapeutic research, the law requires 'full and frank disclosure'. This means adopting a 'reasonable' participant approach and thus telling Michael about the implications of an RCT, its benefits, risks and alternatives. From the brief facts of the case study it seems unlikely that all this information was provided, especially as Michael seems to think he will be taking the new drug. Note too that the consent requirements of the Medicines for Human Use (Clinical Trials) Regulations 2004 have not been complied with (these require consent to be in writing).

The relationship between law and ethics

Similarities between law and ethics

- **Abuse and mistreatment**. The legal and ethical concerns raised by research focus on the same issues: how abuse and mistreatment can be prevented and how a proper balance can be maintained between protecting the rights of the individual and the advancement of science.

- **Independent review**. Both law and ethics recognise the need for independent review of the design and conduct of research to make sure that ethical and legal standards are met.

- **Fundamental rights**. The legal and ethical frameworks regulating research seek to safeguard the same basic rights of participants, namely autonomy, privacy, confidentiality and fair treatment.

Differences between law and ethics

- **Codes/professional guidelines**. In comparison to the numerous codes and professional guidelines regulating research, the law's approach is minimal relying mainly on the common law of consent and Medicine for Human Use (Clinical Trials) Regulations 2004; ethical guidance is also generally much more detailed than the law.

- **Standard of disclosure**. The ethical standard of disclosure is higher than the legal standard, i.e. the law requires less information to be disclosed to participants than is expected to be disclosed in ethical guidance (which generally insists that participants are 'fully informed').

References

Ashcroft, R.E. (2002) An ethical perspective – nursing research. In: *Nursing Law and Ethics*, 2nd edn (eds J. Tingle and A. Cribb). Blackwell Science, Oxford.

British Medical Association (2001)

Campbell, A., Gillett, G. and Jones, G. (2001) *Medical Ethics*, 3rd edn. Oxford University Press, Oxford.

Department of Health (2001) *Governance Arrangements for National Health Service Research Ethics Committees*. HMSO, London.

Department of Health (2004) *Research Governance Framework for Health and Social Care*. HMSO, London.

Foster, C. (2001) *The Ethics of Medical Research on Humans*. Cambridge University Press, Cambridge.

Fox, M. (2002) Clinical research and patients: the legal perspective. In: *Nursing Law and Ethics*, 2nd edn (eds J. Tingle and A. Cribb). Blackwell Science, Oxford.

Hope, T., Savulescu, J. and Hendrick, J. (2003) *Medical Ethics and Law: The core curriculum*. Churchill Livingstone, Edinburgh.

Kennedy, I. and Grubb, A. (2000) *Medical Law*, 3rd edn. Butterworths, London.

Mason, J.K., McCall Smith, R.A. and Laurie, G.T. (2002) *Law and Medical Ethics*, 6th edn. Butterworths, London.

Montgomery, J. (2003) *Health Care Law*. Oxford University Press, Oxford.

Neuberger, J. (1992) *Ethics and Health Care*. King's Fund, London.

Royal College of Nursing (2003) *Research Ethics*. Royal College of Nursing, London.

Stauch, M., Wheat, K. and Tingle, J. (2002) *Sourcebook on Medical Law*, 2nd edn. Cavendish, London.

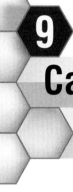

9

Caring for the pregnant woman and the unborn

Learning outcomes

By the end of this chapter you should be able to:

- Discuss the legal and ethical implications of assisted conception
- Consider the scope of a pregnant woman's autonomy
- Assess how genetic medicine can affect reproductive choice
- Evaluate the role of law in regulating pregnancy and childbirth.

⚙━π *Keywords*
....

Reproductive revolution
Describes how assisted conception has introduced a new vocabulary to (and challenged society's traditional attitude to) the family and parenthood

Introduction

The reproductive choices that are now available have made decisions – such as when to have children and in what circumstances – much more complex than they were only a few decades ago. Assisted conception, for example, offers the chance of parenthood to the infertile as well as single women and those living in homosexual relationships. Yet assisted conception, described by many as a '**reproductive revolution**', has not been universally welcomed, especially by those who want to preserve traditional family structures. In examining their objections (and other moral arguments against the various reproductive technologies), this chapter will focus on some of the most hotly debated aspects of reproduction. It will also consider access to treatment and how reproductive choice is affected by developments in genetic medicine. Additionally the scope of a pregnant woman's autonomy will be examined.

Reproductive technologies

In this section we describe the various reproductive technologies (the terms 'assisted conception' and 'reproductive technologies' are used interchangeably), moral arguments against them and how they are regulated, but we begin with a brief definition of infertility.

What is infertility?

There is no objective definition of infertility but the standard medical definition is the failure to conceive after 12 months of regular unprotected sexual intercourse, or the occurrence of three or more miscarriages or stillbirths (Jackson 2001, p. 252). Although it is commonly thought of as a modern social problem, infertility is in fact as old as humanity. But despite its long history, accurate assessments of the extent of infertility are unavailable. That said, it is widely accepted that up to one in seven couples will experience infertility at some point (Human Fertilisation and Embryology Authority 2001). Furthermore, although the debate continues about whether or not infertility is an illness or a disease, justifying its control by doctors, it is undoubtedly true that unwanted childlessness is not only extremely distressing but also threatens people's self-esteem and their sense of control over their lives (McLean 1999, p. 8).

What are the reproductive technologies?

Several techniques are now available. These range from the relatively simple to the more high tech (see box below).

Reproductive technologies

Artificial insemination by husband/partner (AIH/AIP)

Artificial insemination is the oldest technique (first recorded in 1790). It enables sperm to be inserted directly into the cervix via the vagina. Intrauterine insemination (IUI) is essentially the same as AIH but usually combines ovarian stimulation for the woman and preparation of the semen.

Donor insemination (DI)

The first recorded successful DI (sometimes also called artificial insemination by donor, AID) was performed in 1884. It involves the use of sperm from an anonymous donor. It can be used if a husband or partner has no sperm, has few or poor sperm, or risks passing on an inherited disorder. Some clinics offer DI to single women or lesbian couples.

Gamete intrafallopian transfer (GIFT)

In this technique the eggs are collected from the woman, mixed with sperm and then the eggs and sperm are transferred to the fallopian tube before fertilisation takes place. This means that sperm do not have to travel the length of the reproductive canal before encountering an egg. This procedure can use either donated sperm or eggs (or both).

In vitro fertilisation (IVF)

This technique led to the birth of the world's first 'test-tube baby' in 1978. Following hormone stimulation, eggs are collected from a woman and mixed with a man's sperm. Fertilisation occurs in a culture dish. Where appropriate, IVF can also be used with donated eggs, sperm or embryos.

Intracytoplasmic sperm injection (ICSI)

A relatively new technique (first performed successfully in 1999), ICSI involves IVF in which a single sperm is injected directly into each egg to promote the creation of an embryo.

Refle*Reflective activity*

Which reproductive technique described in the box do you think is:

- Most ethically acceptable
- Least ethically acceptable?

What are the moral objections to assisted reproduction?

Keywords

Want society

A society in which it has become fashionable to seek the fulfilment of individual wants and to accept far less readily, if at all, that some desires cannot, should not, or even must not be satisfied

People's moral worries about assisted conception vary greatly. At a very general level it is claimed that assisted conception is morally objectionable because it reflects the rise of the '**want society**'. Other more specific criticisms of assisted conception fall into three broad categories.

Unnaturalness

Those who claim that assisted conception is unnatural use two related arguments. One is that the sacred process of life is up to God and so should not be interfered with. In other words, the infertile should accept their condition as God's will. The other argument is that, since the only natural and legitimate end of sex is procreation, techniques such as IVF and artificial insemination (which sever such a link) are contrary to the natural law (Liu 1991, p. 49).

Although popular, there are three major problems with the 'unnatural' argument. The first is the difficulty of determining what is natural and what is unnatural. The second is that assisted conception is no different from much of modern medicine – which similarly 'interferes with nature' by extending and/or improving people's lives. The third difficulty is that those who rely on the unnatural argument provide no reasons why something that is unnatural is therefore morally wrong. Or, to put it another way, they simply assert that what is 'unnatural' is immoral without explaining why (Warnock 2002, pp. 70–77).

Harm to children – the child welfare argument

Critics of infertility who rely on so-called child welfare arguments are convinced that children will suffer psychological trauma if they are conceived through non-traditional methods (particularly IVF or DI).

The difficulty with this objection is that it assumes (mistakenly) that the circumstances of the birth of such children will be kept secret and that they will therefore never know for certain (but may nevertheless suspect) their origins. Thus the argument – that this deception will blemish, if not destroy, the trust that ideally exists within the family – cannot be sustained (Overall 2002, pp. 305–321).

Feminist arguments

Those who object to assisted conception on 'feminist' grounds take several different approaches. But whatever their particular emphasis they share a conviction that reproductive technologies harm women's physical or mental well-being. Thus, for some the problem concept is 'motherhood' itself. This concept, it is claimed, reinforces the idea that child-rearing is both women's 'natural destiny' and proper role – without which they cannot be completely fulfilled. Or, to put it another way, reproductive technologies degrade women by reinforcing society's expectation that their main function is to become mothers. In short they are 'nothing' unless they bear children.

An alternative feminist approach condemns the way in which infertility treatment takes power over the reproductive process away from women and puts it into the hands of (largely) male medical expertise. This, so it is argued, inevitably means that women's bodies are controlled and manipulated by men for their own (male-dominated) scientific purposes.

Another 'feminist' objection to assisted conception focuses on the effect of infertility treatment. Given the low chance of success for some techniques and their high cost – emotional, physical and financial – it is at least arguable, so critics claim, that assisted conception is not a 'reasonable' choice for many of the childless. This is particularly so given that research suggests that, for a substantial number of women, treatment 'takes over their lives' yet does not provide the peace of mind that it is assumed will come from knowing that they have tried everything (Jackson 2001, p. 178).

The main difficulty with the various feminist objections to assisted conception is they almost always fail to treat the life plans of the infertile with respect. More controversially, in denying the infertile the right to make autonomous decisions they also fail to acknowledge that, for some human beings, having children is of profound importance. So much so, in fact, that it has been argued that procreation is a basic human need – generating moral and legal obligations (on the state) to satisfy that need (Warnock 2002, p. 27; we consider problems of access to treatment below).

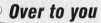

Over to you

Read Hendrick 2000, Chapter 6.

- What are the moral objections to surrogacy?
- How effective is the Surrogacy Arrangements Act 1985?

Regulation of assisted conception

The regulation of reproductive technologies has two principal purposes: first to ensure that the techniques are safe and second to ensure that their use is ethical. Whether the Human Fertilisation and Embryology Act 1990 (the main statute regulating assisted conception) can achieve these two purposes is, however, another matter – not least because the pace of scientific progress is so rapid that the Act suffers from 'in-built obsolescence' (Jackson 2001, p. 185). Thus, although it may have provided a nearly comprehensive scheme for regulating assisted conception when it was first enacted, that is no longer the case. This explains why there have been so many recent challenges to the Act (and why it is currently being reviewed).

The Act basically adopts a threefold approach to regulating assisted conception. This consists of a statutory body – the Human Fertilisation and Embryo Authority – a licensing system and a rigorous consent framework. The main topics covered by the Act are summarised in the box below.

Human Fertilisation and Embryology Act 1990 – main topics

- Establishes a statutory authority (the Human Fertilisation and Embryology Authority)
- Prohibits certain activities
- Enables licences to be issued regulating: a) infertility treatment; b) storage of human eggs, sperm and embryos; and c) research on human embryos
- Defines 'mother' and 'father'
- Regulates disclosure of information and confidentiality
- Provides a defence of conscientious objection
- Gives powers of enforcement and creates criminal offences
- Provides for detailed consent requirements
- Makes provision for a code of practice.

Human Fertilisation and Embryology Authority

The Human Fertilisation and Embryology Authority (HFEA) exists to safeguard, protect and reassure patients, professionals and the public about licensed fertility treatments and human embryo research. Its main statutory functions are to:

- License and regulate clinics that provide treatment and those that carry out research involving human embryos
- Monitor and inspect premises providing treatment
- Publish a code of practice giving guidance to clinics on how they should carry out their activities
- Keep a confidential register of information about donors, patients and treatments
- Give advice and information to people seeking fertility treatment, to donors and to the general public
- Keep the whole field under review.

Licensing system

One of the main ways in which the Act regulates infertility treatment is by prohibiting certain activities altogether (e.g. placing an embryo in an animal, see sections 3 and 4 of the Act). However, it is important to note that not all types of infertility treatment are regulated by the Act. In fact, it is only treatment that involves the creation of an embryo outside a women's body or the use of genetic material that has been donated/stored that falls within the licensing scheme. Thus the main treatments requiring a licence are IVF, DI and GIFT (where donated sperm/eggs are used). Other techniques that are lawful but remain unlicensed are artificial insemination using a husband's or partner's sperm (that has been freshly obtained) and do it yourself techniques – where a woman inseminates herself.

Consent requirements

As regards the law of consent, assisted conception is no different from other medical treatment that involves touching patients. This means that, whether an individual is receiving infertility treatment or providing genetic material (i.e. embryos or gametes), all the essential elements that are required to make consent lawful (Chapter 6) must be present. The HFEA and the Code of Practice (issued by the authority and now in its sixth edition), however, go further than the common law by:

- Specifying that consent must be in writing

Working with the Evidence

IN DEPTH Literature Searching

AIM: To provide a comprehensive overview of the NHS clinical databases and to be able to search these effectively using advanced techniques

23 September 2011	Friday	9am - 12pm
17 October 2011	Monday	1.30 – 4.30pm
04 November 2011	Friday	9am - 12pm
14 February 2012	Tuesday	1.30 – 4.30pm
20 March 2012	Tuesday	9.30am - 12.30pm

The Best Evidence Based Resources

AIM: To understand the purpose and explore the use of prime sources of evidence based information

02 September 2011	Friday	9am - 12pm
14 November 2011	Monday	1.30 - 4.30pm
25 January 2012	Wednesday	9.30am – 12.30pm
01 March 2012	Thursday	1.30 – 4.30pm

Using PubMed Effectively

AIM: To provide an introduction to using PubMed for finding journal articles, including the full text of articles where available

03 October 2011	Monday	9.30am - 12pm
09 December 2011	Friday	9.30am - 12pm
01 February 2012	Wednesday	1.30 - 4pm

To book, call the Library on 0161 419 4690

All courses are free!

Training takes place in Pinewood House, Stepping Hill Hospital

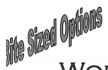

WORKING WITH THE EVIDENCE

BITE SIZED OPTION: Internet for Beginners

AIM: To gain awareness of the range of Internet sites which contain quality health information and to feel confident navigating these sites.

06 September 2011	Tuesday	12 - 1pm
25 November 2011	Friday	9 - 10am
04 January 2012	Wednesday	1 - 2pm
26 March 2012	Monday	4 - 5pm

BITE SIZED OPTION: Literature Searching

AIM: To introduce the clinical databases and learn how to conduct a quick but effective search.

16 September 2011	Friday	9 - 10am
26 October 2011	Wednesday	12 - 1pm
29 November 2011	Tuesday	4 - 5pm
16 December 2011	Friday	9.30 - 10.30am
12 January 2012	Thursday	1 - 2pm
20 February 2012	Monday	2 - 3pm
08 March 2012	Thursday	3 - 4pm

BITE SIZED OPTION: Accessing Full Text Articles

AIM: To be able to access the full text of a journal article from a known reference

11 October 2011	Tuesday	4 - 5pm
09 November 2011	Wednesday	1 - 2pm
17 January 2012	Tuesday	12 - 1pm
16 March 2012	Friday	9 - 10am

TO BOOK, CALL THE LIBRARY ON 0161 419 4690

TRAINING TAKES PLACE IN PINEWOOD HOUSE, STEPPING HILL HOSPITAL

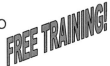

- Providing detailed guidance on the procedure for giving consent (which includes counselling opportunities – see Human Fertilisation and Embryology Authority 2004).

Particularly important too are the rigorous counselling provisions of the Act. These are necessary to ensure that people can make an informed decision especially in relation to ethically sensitive aspects of treatment, such as, for example, the creation of surplus embryos (Lee and Morgan 2001).

Key points | **Top tips**

- The Human Fertilisation and Embryology Authority website at: www.hfea.gov.uk is very comprehensive
- You can download very informative publications about assisted conception, the role of the HFEA, the licensing system, consent requirements and the code of practice

---

Key points | *Top tips*

- The regulation of reproductive technologies consists of three elements: the Human Fertilisation and Embryology Authority, a licensing system and rigorous consent requirements
- The HFEA exists to safeguard, protect and reassure patients, professionals, and the public about licensed infertility treatments and human embryo research

---

Access to treatment – does everyone have a 'right' to reproduce

Moral issues

Before we can answer the question 'Does everyone have a right to reproduce?', we need to realise that the phrase 'right to reproduce' can be interpreted in several different ways. These are: the right to have one's own biological children (whether by natural or artificial means); the right to be a 'social' parent, in other words to rear and found a family (e.g. as a foster parent); or the right to choose to reproduce. That said there can be no doubt that many regard the desire for children as a basic need and a fundamental moral and human right (Warnock 2002, p. 27). This explains why the importance of the family unit is recognised in various international declarations of human rights and the Human Rights Act 1998 (Article 12). Taken together these documents arguably do recognise a moral right to procreate, even though the extent of this right has yet to be determined.

Nor is it yet clear whether the 'rights' recognised imply a positive right to have a child. Indeed, as Kennedy and Grubb point out (2000), international documents on human rights could be interpreted as only protecting a right to choose whether or not to reproduce rather than an absolute right to do so.

Legal issues

As far as the law is concerned, case law to date suggests that the courts are unlikely to recognise the right to reproduce as an absolute legal right (*R.* v. *Secretary of State for the Home Department ex p. Mellor* [2001]). But the main legal issue in this context is about access to infertility treatment – which turns on one of the most questionable sections in the 1990 Act: the so-called 'welfare' provision in section 13(5). The section is very short (and very vague). It states that '*a woman shall not be provided with treatment unless account has been taken of any child who may be born as a result of the treatment (including the need of that child for a father), and of any other child who may be affected by the birth*'.

To help clinics interpret this welfare provision the code of practice (Human Fertilisation and Embryology Authority 2004) gives guidance on the factors they should consider when selecting people for treatment. These include:

● Their commitment to having and bringing up a child (or children)
● Their ability to provide a stable and supportive environment
● Their medical histories and health and future ability to look after a child.

The code also stresses that no category of woman should be excluded from treatment. Much has been written about how clinics should apply the welfare provision (e.g. Jackson 2001, pp. 192–197). But, because decisions are made on a case-by-case basis, there are wide regional differences in the way clinics interpret the section. There is also strong evidence that doctors (and others involved in the assessment and selection process) have too wide a discretion – to reject people they consider medically unsuitable or (more controversially) those they deem unsuitable or unfit to be parents.

So what legal remedies are available to women who have been refused treatment? Few cases have reached the courts on this issue.

There is no doubt, however, that decisions made by clinics cannot be legally challenged unless they are irrational (Montgomery 2003, p. 493, see further *R* v. *Ethical Committee of St Mary's Hospital ex p. Harriott* [1988] and *R* v. *Sheffield HA ex p. Seale* [1996]). What is considered irrational is, needless to say, somewhat unclear.

ꜟꜟꜟ*Reflective activity*

Which of the following categories would you reject as potential parents? Why?
- A single person
- A postmenopausal woman aged 55
- A couple, one of whom has had a previous voluntary sterilisation
- A lesbian couple
- A couple whose only child has died
- A woman who has previously worked as a prostitute.

Over to you

Access the National Institute for Clinical Excellence website at: www.nice.org.uk/cgo11. Critically reflect on recommendations it made (in February 2004) about infertility treatment.

Controlling pregnant women

Moral aspects – does a pregnant woman have moral obligations to her foetus?

There is now clear evidence of what is 'good for' a foetus, i.e. what will most promote its health and development and what prenatal factors (social, environmental and economic) are linked with future ill health. Does that mean, therefore, that if you are pregnant you have a moral obligation to follow all available medical (and other) advice, so as to avoid any possible risk, however remote, to the foetus?

To some the answer to this question is clear. If a pregnant woman neglects her own health by, for example, abusing drugs, smoking or drinking excessively (or ignores advice about diet and lifestyle), the potential hazards of which are now well documented – then in so far as these risks are unnecessary and unreasonable it is at least arguable that she is morally at fault. But for others the answer is less clear-cut. Thus they may concede that pregnant women have a moral duty to at least consider the impact of their behaviour on the developing foetus. Yet to go further than that and assert that, as a consequence, they have a moral responsibility to lead a healthy prenatal lifestyle (McLean 1999) is a step too far.

The reasons they give for limiting the moral responsibility of pregnant women are as follows.

Autonomy/privacy

Constraining a pregnant woman's behaviour would infringe her autonomy and right not to have her body invaded or even touched without consent. Many constraints on her behaviour would involve such a battery (Hope *et al.* 2003, p. 124).

Variable standard of behaviour

The burgeoning literature – some of which is contradictory – and the uncertainty as to what is 'safe' during pregnancy, together with the wide variations in the quality of antenatal care (and access to it), make it unlikely that an appropriate standard of behaviour could be agreed. Furthermore, as Brazier points out (1999) it would be both unreasonable and unfair to impose the same standards on all women irrespective of the differences in their lives and the fact that their ability to take care of themselves depends on personal circumstances, such as their education.

Public policy

The likely consequences of allowing foetal interests to take priority (over a pregnant woman's) is unacceptable in a liberal society. This is because it could lead to pregnant women being imprisoned or impoverished for behaviour that would be tolerated in men or in women who were not pregnant.

Individual versus collective responsibility

Health promotion advice and preventative health programmes concerned with foetal health typically target pregnant women with advice about the steps they should take to ensure the birth of a healthy baby. As a consequence other factors such as, for example, poverty, inadequate social care and environmental toxins (which can potentially have a much more significant harmful impact on foetal development) are neglected. In other words, society's collective responsibility for foetal health (i.e. the social causes of disease) is unfairly shifted to pregnant women themselves (Jackson 2001, p. 159).

Legal aspects of pregnancy – what legal duties do pregnant women owe to the foetus?

In this section we consider whether pregnant women have legal duties towards their unborn children, in particular whether they are liable for injuries to the foetus and whether the law can be used to control their behaviour while pregnant. Before looking at these issues, however, we need to outline the most important case in this context, *Re F* (1988). The case involved a local authority which tried to make a foetus a ward of court so that it would be protected from its mother – a 36-year-old woman with long-standing mental health problems who was abusing drugs and leading a nomadic life.

If successful, these proceedings would have required the mother to live in a specified place and attend hospital. The court rejected the local authority's application and decided that, until it was born (and had a separate existence from its mother), a foetus was not a legal person. In other words, in legal terms it was not a person in its own right.

The effect of *Re F* does not mean that the foetus has no legal protection at all (see Chapter10). Nevertheless it does have two significant legal consequences affecting:

- The liability of mothers for injuries to their foetus
- The role of law in regulating the behaviour of pregnant women.

Mothers' legal liability for injuries to the foetus

Briefly, the effect of *Re F* is that generally (the main exception being in respect of injuries caused by negligent driving) mothers cannot be sued by their children for injuries sustained during pregnancy – even though they may have caused those injuries (e.g. through drug addiction and so on). As we shall see, they may, however, be able to sue someone else (see also Chapter 10).

There are two main reasons for this maternal immunity, i.e. why English law exempts mothers from liability for prenatal injury (and so treats pregnant women who injure a foetus differently from everyone else). First, it would have a harmful effect on family life if mothers had to pay compensation to their disabled babies and children. Second, given the very different personal and social circumstances of pregnant woman it would be very difficult, if not impossible, for the law to set an appropriate standard of care, i.e. one that a 'reasonable' pregnant woman would be legally required to meet. The difficulty of setting acceptable legal standards of care also (at least in part) explains why the law's role in regulating the behaviour of pregnant women is so limited.

The role of law in controlling behaviour during pregnancy

In considering the role of law in controlling pregnant women's behaviour we are really asking whether they can be legally restrained (or punished) from acting in a way that may harm the foetus. Currently, such legal intervention is unlawful. There are several reasons for this approach.

First, there would be enormous practical difficulties in enforcing any legal restriction. It would mean, for example, that pregnant women would have to be kept under almost constant surveillance until they gave birth. Second, any gains to foetal health (which might well be marginal) would be won at much too high a cost – in other words, at the expense of pregnant women's legal right to bodily integrity and privacy. Third, imposing any legal restrictions on how pregnant women behaved would risk turning health professionals into police informers (Mason *et al.* 2002, p. 422). And finally there is the very real possibility that, fearing prosecution (or some other legal consequence), pregnant women would not seek medical help at all – which might endanger the foetus even more.

Key points *Top tips*

- The foetus has no legal rights of its own until it is born
- The foetus cannot sue its mother for injuries caused *in utero*
- The law does not restrict women's behaviour during pregnancy

---

Prenatal genetic testing

Currently the proportion of childhood deaths attributable wholly or partly to genetic factors is about 50% (Mason *et al.* 2002, p. 184). And, as it becomes increasingly clear that there is a genetic component in many illnesses and conditions, the value of **prenatal genetic testing** cannot be exaggerated. But despite the enormous reproductive choice prenatal testing can offer would-be parents, it does raise several fundamental ethical issues. In this final section we look briefly at some of these issues, but first we need to define what prenatal testing involves.

What is prenatal genetic testing?

Prenatal genetic testing is used to investigate individual pregnancies where the foetus, because of a specified reason such as

⚷ Keywords

Prenatal genetic testing
Testing pregnant women where the foetus is considered to be at increased risk of a genetic disorder

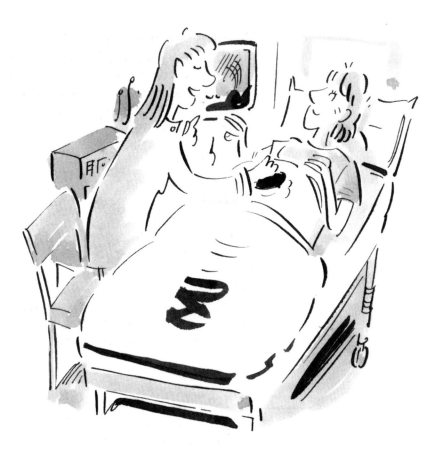

Prenatal genetic testing.

maternal age, family history or a positive screening test, is judged to be at an increased risk of a genetic condition. The main groups of women who are likely to have prenatal testing are those where there is a positive family history (and thus a high risk of a problem recurring) and those where there is an increased risk without a family history (e.g. the increased risk of Down's syndrome for older mothers).

There are various kinds of prenatal test. These include amniocentesis, chorionic villus sampling (CVS) and foetal blood sampling as well as diagnostic ultrasound and laboratory techniques (e.g. chromosome analysis) The conditions tested for include chromosome disorders (e.g. Down's syndrome), mutations in single genes (e.g. Huntington's disease, cystic fibrosis, sickle cell disease) and structural malformations. Whatever test is carried out the intention is either to confirm or to exclude the presence in a foetus of a specific genetic disorder. In some cases, however, the results may be less than definite and other tests may be required.

Top tips

The main purposes of prenatal diagnosis are:

● To inform and prepare parents for the birth of an affected infant
● To allow *in utero* treatment or delivery at a specialist centre for immediate postnatal treatment
● To allow termination of an affected foetus

What ethical issues does prenatal genetic testing raise?

Ethical concerns about prenatal testing range from the effects on individuals to broader social effects (Alderson 2002, p. 197). They include the following.

The rights and wrongs of abortion

If the only option available to prevent a child being born with a genetic disease is a termination of the pregnancy, the ethical questions commonly raised in debates about abortion become central. These focus on the moral status of the foetus, in particular whether it has a right to life and when life begins (see Chapter 10).

What conditions should be tested for – the spectre of 'designer babies'

It is genetic testing's potential for misuse that most causes concern. Thus, normally, abortion (or embryo selection) following genetic testing is limited, i.e. carried out to prevent the birth of a baby with a 'significant disability or abnormality' associated with, for example, chromosomal abnormalities (i.e. Down's syndrome) or gene mutations (such as cystic fibrosis or Duchenne's muscular dystrophy) (Hope *et al.* 2003). But the increasing sophistication of genetic information and medicine raises fears about how far society could go in defining abnormality. In other words, do the new reproductive technologies encourage people to want only 'perfect' babies – resembling a consumer commodity – rather than a valued person with ordinary human failings (Alderson 2002, p. 198)? The fear is, in short, that prenatal screening will not just be used to prevent debilitating genetic disease and disability but will enable prospective parents to 'play God', creating 'designer babies (i.e. those that fit society's idea of 'normal').

Discrimination against the disabled

But what is the distinction between normal and abnormal? According to those who are keen to promote the equal treatment of disabled people, prenatal genetic testing is harmful because it presupposes that there is such a distinction, in other words that normality is a 'fact' that can be objectively defined. But the disability lobby rejects this assumption. They claim that what we think of as abnormal is much more subjective. Accordingly it will be influenced by many factors (such as our personal experiences) as well as by a particular society's attitudes to disability. Using prenatal testing to prevent disabled people being born simply reinforces society's uncaring and discriminatory attitude to the disabled. Rather than concentrating efforts on eliminating 'abnormal' foetuses, therefore, society should provide better services for the disabled and cater for their special needs.

Key points ~~Top tips~~

- Prenatal genetic tests aim to detect genetic abnormalities
- Ethical issues raised by prenatal testing include the morality of abortion, 'designer babies' and discrimination against the disabled

What legal issues does prenatal testing raise?

The legal issues raised by prenatal testing focus mainly on the law of consent (see Chapter 6). In brief testing is lawful if consent is obtained. In particular this means that patients must be given full information about:

- The condition(s) being tested for
- The nature of the proposed testing procedure
- Its scope and limitations
- Risks associated with the tests
- The accuracy, potential implications and use of the result.

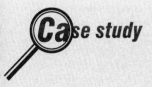
Case study

Can Betsy be forced to have a caesarean?

Betsy is 38 weeks pregnant. On her last antenatal visit she was advised that a caesarean section was almost certainly going to be necessary. Betsy is very unhappy about this advice – she has always wanted a natural birth (as her birth plan records). A few hours ago Betsy was rushed into hospital, as her labour is well under way. As anticipated, however, it soon becomes clear that without a caesarean Betsy's life and that of her baby are at risk. Nevertheless, Betsy is adamant. She will not have a caesarean.

You are very worried by Betsy's decision.

Case study continued

ꜱꙅ·ᴙ*Reflective activity*

1. What moral dilemmas are raised by Betsy's refusal of treatment?
2. Can she be legally forced to have a caesarean?

1. Moral dilemmas

The central moral dilemma raised by forced caesareans is that, on the one hand, a situation in which doctors idly stand by and allow a mature foetus to rupture its mother's womb arguably does serious damage to the concept of the sanctity of life, which any society must maintain. On the other hand, the thought that doctors could carry out invasive and potentially risky treatment on unwilling patients is deeply troubling to the concept of individual autonomy, another of liberal society's fundamental values (Stauch *et al.* 2002, p. 480).

The main moral argument in favour of forced caesareans asserts that a mother-to-be has a natural duty and moral obligation to do all that is reasonably possible to ensure that her baby is safely delivered. This duty arises because of the 'special relationship' between mother and child. In other words, just as pregnancy imposes special moral obligations on women so does the voluntary act of continuing a pregnancy to term create special obligations over and above those that are normally expected. Applying this argument to Betsy means that she is morally responsible for the life within her and so must do all she can to ensure its well-being, i.e. have a caesarean.

The main moral argument against forced caesareans relies on the value our society places on autonomy. In Betsy's situation this means the right she alone has to decide what medical treatment to accept or refuse. Those who rely on the autonomy argument assume, of course, that autonomy is an absolute value and so does not have to be balanced against other important values, such as the life and health of the 'nearly born' foetus.

2. Legal considerations

A spate of high-profile cases in the 1990s (e.g. *Re M B* [1997]) established beyond any doubt that, providing a pregnant woman is competent, she has the absolute legal right to refuse all treatment – even if that means that she and/or the foetus will die or be seriously harmed. Furthermore, this legal right exists even if 'her thinking process was unusual, bizarre, irrational and contrary to the overwhelming majority of the community at large' (*Re St George's Health Care NHS Trust* v. *S* [1999]).

But what if Betsy is not competent? This is an important question, because then health professionals can act in her best interests (and so can carry out any procedure, including a caesarean). Much will therefore depend on the assessment of Betsy's competence. However, as many commentators (e.g. Jackson 2001, Brazier 1997) have pointed out, in practice it may be all too easy for health professionals to question a woman's competence given the effect of shock, fatigue, confusion, panic, pain and drugs (all of which the courts have suggested can cause temporary incompetence but which are nevertheless an inevitable part of childbirth).

In summary, then, if health professionals decide Betsy is not competent they can ignore her wishes and do what they think is in her best interests. This will normally include saving her life or preventing serious harm. It will inevitably also include doing everything necessary to enable her to give birth to a live baby.

Reflective activity

Do you think that Betsy has a moral obligation to undergo a caesarean? Explain your answer. Compare it with a colleague's.

The relationship between law and ethics

Similarities between law and ethics

- The legal and moral framework regulating pregnancy, assisted conception and genetic testing seek to reconcile potentially conflicting interests, i.e. those of society as a whole, the foetus, would-be-parents and individual families.

- The legal and ethical principles underpinning genetic testing seek to protect the autonomy and confidentiality of those involved.

- For genetic testing to be lawful and ethical rigorous consent requirements must be met; these emphasise how consent must be fully informed.

- The code of practice (issued by the HFEA) regulating assisted conception reinforces legal principles, in particular the need for informed consent and effective counselling.

Differences between law and ethics

- In regulating access to assisted conception, the law places the interest of the 'future' child at centre-stage – Human Fertilisation and Embryology Act 1990, section 13(5); ethical considerations, on the other hand, emphasise the rights of would-be-parents.

- In recognising the right of competent pregnant women to refuse medical treatment (*Re M.B.* [1997]) the law clearly places the autonomy of the woman above any moral interests of the foetus.

- In exempting mothers from liability for injuries caused to the foetus, the law fails to protect any moral claims it may have (e.g. to a 'healthy' environment in which to develop).

- Although the moral claims of the foetus are widely recognised, the law does not restrict women's behaviour during pregnancy.

Rapid recap

Check your progress so far by working through each of the following questions.

1. What is the role of the Human Fertilisation and Embryology Authority?
2. The regulation of assisted conception has two main purposes: what are they?
3. What is the main aim of prenatal genetic testing?
4. What does the phrase 'maternal immunity' mean?
5. Can a competent pregnant woman be forced to have a caesarean?

If you have difficulty with more than one of the questions, read through the section again to refresh your understanding before moving on.

References

Alderson, P. (2002) Prenatal counselling and images of disability. In: *Ethical Issues in Maternal–Foetal Medicine* (ed. D.L. Dickenson). Cambridge University Press, Cambridge.

Brazier, M. (1997) Parental responsibilities, foetal welfare and children's welfare. In: *Family Law Towards the Millennium* (ed. C. Bridge). Butterworths, London.

Hendrick, J. (2000) *Law and Ethics in Nursing and Health Care*. Stanley Thornes, Cheltenham.

Hope, T., Savulescu, J. and Hendrick, J. (2003) *Medical Ethics and Law: The core curriculum*. Churchill Livingstone, Edinburgh.

Human Fertilisation and Embryology Authority (2004) *Code of Practice*, 6th edn. HFEA, London.

Jackson, E. (2001) *Regulating Reproduction: Law, technology and autonomy*. Hart, Oxford.

Kennedy, I. and Grubb, A. (2000) *Medical Law*, 3rd edn. Butterworths, London.

Lee, R.G. and Morgan, D. (2001) *Human Fertilisation and Embryology: Regulating the reproductive revolution*. Blackstone Press, London.

Liu, A. (1991) *Artificial Reproduction and Reproductive Rights*. Dartmouth, Aldershot.

McLean, S. (1999) *Old Law, New Medicine: Medical ethics and human rights*. Pandora, London.

Mason, J.K., McCall Smith, R.A. and Laurie, G.T. (2002) *Law and Medical Ethics*, 6th edn. Butterworths, London.

Montgomery, J. (2003) *Health Care Law*. Oxford University Press, Oxford.

Overall, C. (2002) Do new reproductive technologies benefit or harm children? In: *Ethical Issues in Maternal–Foetal Medicine* (ed. D.L. Dickenson). Cambridge University Press, Cambridge.

Stauch, M., Wheat, K. and Tingle, J. (2002) *Sourcebook on Medical Law*, 2nd edn. Cavendish, London.

Warnock, M. (2002) *Making Babies: Is there a right to have children?* Oxford University Press, Oxford.

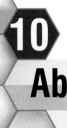

10

Abortion, sterilisation and birth control

Learning outcomes

By the end of this chapter you should be able to:

- Understand the ethical and legal issues raised by abortion
- Assess the ethical and legal implications of sterilisation
- Discuss the legal regulation of birth control.

Introduction

Although abortion is no longer the 'hottest' moral dilemma in health-care ethics it continues to arouse passionate disagreement. This is so even though the Abortion Act, which liberalised abortion, was passed almost 40 years ago. In looking at the rights and wrongs of abortion this chapter considers some of the most difficult questions in the debate – such as: Whose life is more important: the mother's or the child's? and When does life begin?

As regards sterilisation (in particular non-consensual sterilisation), this topic has been chosen because the impact of the Human Rights Act 1998 means that we can no longer ignore the rights of people who, in the past, might all too easily have been prevented from reproducing. Thus, while the decision to sterilise an incompetent woman might relatively recently have prompted few concerns, that is no longer the case. In other words, now that many regard the right to reproduce as a basic human right there have to be very good reasons to sterilise a woman without her consent. This chapter considers what those reasons are, i.e. the moral and legal issues raised by non-voluntary sterilisation. The chapter ends with a brief outline of the legality of various methods of birth control.

Abortion

Abortion is almost certainly the oldest and most common operation for women of reproductive age (Tschudin 2003, p. 125). Approximately 186 000 abortions are carried out each year in England and Wales (about 17 women per 1000 of reproductive age have an abortion). Yet, despite being so commonplace, arguments about the rights and wrongs of abortion continue to rage. There are two main reasons for the continuing debate. First, abortion raises profoundly important questions – such as the moral and legal status

🔑 *Keywords*

Foetus
The term used to describe the developing human being from 6 weeks gestation to the time of birth

of the **foetus** and what it means to be a person. Secondly, advances in medical technology, better diagnostic procedures and more sophisticated genetic tests now enable much more to be known about the foetus than was possible in the past.

Because it is common to hear abortion discussed in terms of rights of the foetus, the mother and other interested parties, a similar approach will be taken here.

Foetal rights

What is the moral status of the foetus?

At the heart of the debate around abortion is the question of the moral status of the foetus. Several different positions can be taken on this. Here are some.

🔑 *Keywords*

Right to life
The view that the foetus has the same moral claims as a person and thus the right not to be deliberately killed

Right to life – life begins at conception

The **right to life** (or pro-life) argument asserts that the embryo and foetus have the same moral status as a human being and therefore the same right to life as any other human being. It is based on the religious belief that life is sacrosanct and thus that God alone has the authority both to give life and to take it away. This sanctity of life doctrine is often summed up in the following way: it is wrong to kill innocent human beings; a human foetus is an innocent human being; therefore it is wrong to kill a human foetus.

This view of abortion is usually described as conservative. It is underpinned by the belief that there is a specific moment when life begins, namely at conception (when the sperm and egg come together). It is at this point that the embryo acquires the same full moral status as a human being.

🔑 *Keywords*

Embryo
Usually understood to describe the developing human being from fertilisation to 6 weeks gestation

A more moderate view of abortion challenges this 'early' acquisition of moral status claiming that even though the **embryo** (at this very early stage) is genetically human (i.e. it has the physical existence of a 'being', recognisable as a member of the species Homo Sapiens), it does not have a right to life because it lacks the characteristics that qualify it as a person Essentially therefore this argument asserts that only when the foetus becomes a **person** does it have full moral rights or indeed any moral rights at all.

🔑 *Keywords*

Person
A human being that has certain identifiable capacities and characteristics (the term is often used interchangeably with 'human being')

Personhood – when is a person a person?

According to the personhood approach certain essential capacities or characteristics (normally associated with being a person) are so morally important that they justify treating such a creature differently from (and valuing it more than) all others, such as animals or fish. The main difficulty with this approach is that not only are there several personhood theories but few philosophers agree on how a 'proper' person can be identified (i.e. what capacities or characteristics an entity must have to achieve personhood status). Here are just some of those that have been suggested (e.g. see Warren 1997; Tooley 1983; Harris 1985):

- **Emotionality**: the capacity to feel happy, sad, angry, loving, etc.
- **Self-awareness** (also called self-consciousness): being capable of valuing one's own existence, having some sense of one's own identity and being able to imagine the future
- **Communication**: the capacity to communicate (by whatever means)
- **Moral agency**: the capacity to regulate one's own actions through moral principles and ideals and so be held accountable, praised and blamed
- **Reasoning**: the capacity to make decisions and solve new and relatively complex problems
- **Sentience**: the capacity to feel pain or pleasure
- **Sense of justice**: this includes an awareness of what it is to have a 'right'.

With such a wide choice of characteristics or capacities (but little agreement on the one(s) that is/are essential to personhood) it is not surprising that many philosophers have abandoned the idea that you can pinpoint the absolute moment at which a person materialises (and so has a moral status). Glover (1990), for example, argues that being a person may not have sharp boundaries at all. So, just as there is no single moment when you become middle-aged, similarly there is no absolute point when you develop the distinctive characteristics of personhood. This approach is called the gradualist position.

The gradualist position

Simply put, the gradualist position asserts that you cannot draw a line and say 'before this point the thing is not a person, after this point it is a person'. Rather, the claim is that humanity is a quality that develops with time (Mason 1998, p. 110). In other words, the foetus has some moral status but not as much as it has at birth. Consequently, as the pregnancy develops so the moral worth of the foetus increases (as does its entitlement to more of our respect) until it reaches birth – at which time it acquires the same full moral status as a person.

If you accept the gradualist position, then the justification for abortion will have to become stronger as the foetus matures. As we shall see, this gradualist approach is basically how the law treats the foetus – as a moral entity that possess different (and greater) rights as it moves towards birth.

Reflective activity

Which approach to the moral status of the foetus do you find most convincing? Why?

Key points | Top tips

- Anti-abortionists who adopt the most 'conservative' pro-life position object to abortion on religious grounds, i.e. the sanctity of life doctrine
- Some anti-abortionists object to abortion because of the potential of the foetus to become a 'person'

What is the legal status of the foetus?

As we saw in Chapter 9, English law does not recognise the foetus as a legal person (*Re F* [1988]). In short it is not a person in its own right. What this means is that it is only after birth, i.e. once a baby is born alive and has a separate existence from its mother, that any legal action can be brought on its behalf. But despite its lack of legal status, the foetus does have some legal protection before birth. For example:

- **Criminal law**. If the foetus is harmed *in utero* as a result of a criminal act committed against its mother then, providing it is born alive, the perpetrator can face criminal charges. This happened in *Attorney-General's Reference (no. 3 of 1994)* (1997). The case concerned a pregnant woman who was stabbed and gave birth to a premature baby 2 weeks later (at 26 weeks). The child survived for 120 days (dying because she was premature rather than from the injuries caused by the assault). The accused was nevertheless found guilty of manslaughter. Note also that deliberate non-treatment of a living **abortus** might result in murder or manslaughter charges.

- **Tort law**. Under the Congenital Disabilities (Civil Liability) Act 1976 a foetus can sue for certain pre-birth injuries if it is born alive. In one 2001 case, for example, a girl aged 8 received £2.43

Keywords

Abortus

A human foetus whose weight is less than 0.5 kilograms when removed or expelled from the mother's body

million under the Act for injuries she sustained when she was stabbed in the head with an amniocentesis needle while a foetus of 16 weeks. She was profoundly brain-damaged as a result (Dimond 2002, p. 272). The 1976 Act is complex and is summarised in the box below.

Main aspects of the Congenital Civil Disabilities Act 1976

The child can sue:

- if it is born alive (it must survive for at least 48 hours)
- for harm caused by negligent action to the father or mother
- which resulted in the child being born disabled.

Other points to note:

- Disability is widely defined as 'any deformity, disease or abnormality, including predisposition to physical or mental defect in the future'
- Liability generally does not arise if the parents knew of the risk of the child being born disabled
- The mother is not liable to the child (unless the injuries to the foetus were caused while she was driving)
- Where a parent is partly to blame for the child's disabilities, compensation can be reduced to take account of his/her share of the responsibility.

Various other legal provisions also go some way towards protecting the future interests of the foetus. Thus parents' behaviour during pregnancy might, for example, prompt care proceedings, with the result that as soon as a baby is born it is taken into care by social workers. This happened in *Re D* [1987], where both parents were drug addicts (and the mother continued to take drugs while pregnant).

In summary, then, it is clear that, despite the foetus's lack of legal status *in utero*, it does nevertheless have some legal rights (albeit only if born alive).

Key points | Top tips

There are several types of pre-birth injuries that a child born disabled can sue for under the 1976 Act. These include:

- Negligent genetic counselling and prenatal testing
- Negligent infertility treatment
- Preconception injuries (e.g. exposure to chemicals or excessive radiation)
- Injuries during pregnancy (e.g. those caused by drugs negligently prescribed, developed or manufactured)
- Injuries during birth (e.g. negligent delivery procedures).

- Although the foetus is not a legal person, after it is born action can be taken on its behalf
- Under the Congenital Disabilities (Civil Liability) Act 1976 a child can sue for injuries caused before its birth

Maternal rights

Moral aspects

In this section we focus on what is usually called 'the pro-choice lobby'. It is described as feminist because it regards pregnancy as a uniquely female experience that must be controlled by the individual woman concerned and not by others. But, as Whyte points out (1997, p. 16), unlike the anti-abortionists, who can usually easily express their message in sound-bites (such as abortion is killing, killing is bad, abortion is bad), the pro-abortion lobby have much more complex arguments to get across – not just the right of a woman to decide but also 'a tangle of moral, personal and social factors'. Those who claim that a woman's right to control her own body is one of the most basic of human rights typically rely on a variety of 'rights' to support their approach. Briefly these are as follows.

Right to self-defence

If you use the self-defence argument you are basically saying that you have a right to defend yourself against an intruder who threatens you in some way (McDonagh 2002). Most commonly used when pregnancy threatens the mother's life, few (except perhaps ultraconservatives) would deny that the mother's right to life comes first and overrides any right the foetus may have not to be deliberately killed. Similarly, if the mother is raped the self-defence argument is very persuasive (likewise if she is diagnosed with an illness treatment for which poses a risk to the foetus). But in some cases where the risk to the mother's physical or mental health is less serious, the self-defence argument becomes harder to justify.

Autonomy

In their most extreme form autonomy arguments assert that women have the right to self-determination and liberty. This means that they have the right to decide what is to happen to their body, in particular to decide not to continue with a pregnancy – at whatever stage and for whatever reason, however trivial. Some supporters of the autonomy argument also claim that, because pregnancy is a risky undertaking (even when voluntary), to deny a woman an abortion infringes her right to physical integrity and freedom from bodily harm (Warren 1993).

A variant of the autonomy argument is based on the idea that a woman has rights to ownership of her body. What this essentially means is that she has the right to reject any 'occupant' she is unwilling to shelter. It is only, therefore, if a woman has accepted special responsibility for a foetus – by, for example, not trying to prevent its existence – that she is obliged to continue with the pregnancy. If, on the other hand she has used all reasonable contraceptive precautions, then she cannot be assumed to have accepted responsibility for the unwelcome foetus, who accordingly has no right of occupation (Thomson 1971).

Consequences for the future

There is ample evidence throughout history that, without access to safe, effective and accessible abortions, women will resort to back-street abortionists (almost always unqualified) or folk remedies. Either way they put their health at risk and some will die. Indeed, current research suggests that, out of the quarter of the world's population who live in countries where abortion is either illegal or very restricted, at least 20 million women a year have illegal abortions, resulting in nearly 80 000 deaths (Jackson 2001). Nor are the consequences of forcing women to continue with unwanted pregnancies any more acceptable. Not only will they have too many children – thus facing the risks of pregnancy and the perils of childbirth – but their choices following birth may be very limited (Warren 1993).

Key points Top tips

- 'Feminist' arguments supporting 'a woman's right to choose' are usually described as 'pro-choice'
- The rights on which the pro-choice lobby rely are: a) autonomy, b) self-defence and c) consequences for the future

---

Legal aspects

Before looking at the Abortion Act 1967 two important points (which are often overlooked) need to be stressed. These are:

- Although generally characterised as a permissive statute, the Act offers the foetus some protection (by, for example, limiting 'late' abortions) but at the same time denies it full legal personhood
- Because access to abortion is controlled by doctors (see below) it can be seen as putting into place a subtle system of medical control over women's fertility rather than giving them the right to control their own reproductive autonomy.

The Act is widely described as a compromise measure. This is because it failed to satisfy the demands of those who wanted 'abortion on demand' but at the same time was attacked by pro-life campaigners as conceding too much.

Women's rights under the Abortion Act 1967

Access to abortion – does the Act give women a legal right to abortion?

It is a mistake to think that women have a legal right to abortion, since the Act does not entitle them to demand an abortion, even during the early stages of pregnancy. Instead, it gives doctors the right to decide whether a woman's particular circumstances meet the terms for an abortion specified in the Act (in effect this gives doctors a 'gate-keeping' role).

When is an abortion legal?

Abortions are legal provided they are performed by a registered medical practitioner after two registered medical practitioners have decided 'in good faith' that one or more of the grounds specified in the Act apply. These are summarised in the box below.

The Abortion Act 1967

- **The social ground**: to avoid adverse effects, albeit relatively minor ones to the woman's physical or mental health or that of her family. Abortions in this category (which account for approximately 96% of all abortions) can only be performed if the pregnancy has not exceeded its 24th week.
- **The preventive ground**: to prevent grave permanent injury to he physical or mental health of the pregnant woman. There is no definition in the Act of the word 'permanent'.
- **The life-saving ground**: this ground is very limited as there has to be a risk of death before it can be invoked.
- **The foetal disability ground**: to prevent the birth of 'seriously handicapped' infants. Approximately 1% of abortions are performed on this ground. The Act gives no guidance about how terms such as 'serious handicap' should be interpreted.

continued

Other points to note:

- Except in emergencies (i.e. when an abortion is necessary to save the mother's life or prevent grave permanent injury to her physical or mental health) abortions have to be performed in NHS hospitals or other 'approved' places (e.g. private clinics)
- The Act gives health professionals who carry out abortions according to the Act immunity from prosecution – it does not decriminalise abortion in general
- Nursing staff who, for example, administer prostaglandin infusions are acting lawfully providing they are acting under the instructions of a doctor.

Other people's rights

The father

There has been a steady trickle of cases in the English courts where 'fathers' have attempted to prevent their partners from having an abortion. None has been successful. From these cases it is clear that English law gives fathers no rights to challenge or veto an abortion. Nor do they have the right to be consulted or informed that an abortion has been performed.

Health professionals – can you refuse to participate in an abortion?

Except in an emergency (when an abortion is necessary to save a woman's life or prevent her grave permanent injury) you can refuse to participate in an abortion. This is because the Act has a 'conscience' clause that allows you to do what otherwise would amount to a breach of your contract of employment. If you want to rely on the conscience clause, however, you should declare your objection as soon as you can after you start your employment.

Reflective activity

Do you think the Abortion Act strikes the right balance between the 'rights' of the foetus and those of pregnant women who wish to end their pregnancies? Do you think some abortions are morally 'worse' than others? If so, why?

Key points Top tips

- An abortion is illegal unless one or more grounds specified in the Act apply
- Except in emergencies you can refuse to take part in an abortion

Sterilisation

As was noted in the introduction, the focus of this section is non-voluntary **sterilisation**. But we begin by distinguishing between voluntary and non-voluntary sterilisation.

⊶ₙ Keywords

Sterilisation
The aim of sterilisation (which is generally intended to be permanent) is to end a person's ability to reproduce

Voluntary sterilisation

In voluntary sterilisation the patient is competent and so is able to consent to the procedure.

Moral aspects

Moral worries about voluntary sterilisation usually focus on the fact that the person may later change his/her mind (but may not be able to have the sterilisation reversed). Indeed, despite being the most commonly used method of birth control worldwide, research suggests that it is the permanence of sterilisation and the high level of regret it causes that is its main drawback (Jackson 2001, p. 19). Other moral objections to sterilisation focus on the fear that the social and personal pressures a person may be under when they seek treatment could result in his/her consent not being 'real'.

Legal aspects

There is no doubt that voluntary sterilisation is lawful – providing, of course, that consent has been obtained (see Chapter 6). It is clear too that there is no legal requirement to inform a person's spouse or partner of the procedure.

Non-voluntary sterilisation – in cases of incapacity

We use the phrase non-voluntary sterilisation to describe cases where the patient is incompetent and so cannot consent.

Moral aspects

Sterilising a patient without her consent is undoubtedly one of the most controversial forms of non-consensual treatment. That it raises profound legal and moral concerns is beyond doubt even though many regard it as the only way that some intellectually disabled women will be able to live in the community and have fulfilling relationships. The most common moral concerns about non-voluntary sterilisation are:

◉━🔑 Keywords

Eugenics
The belief that mental capacity and behaviour can be genetically determined and so can be eliminated by selective sterilisation

Eugenics

Those who object to the **eugenics** approach consider it immoral because it hides the 'real' (but unexpressed) reason behind non-voluntary sterilisation – to prevent the patient's condition being passed on (thereby improving the 'human race'). Or, to put it more starkly, the aim is to make sure the 'unfit' or 'defective' do not reproduce. What haunts objectors, in short, is the spectre of compulsory sterilisation programmes – usually associated with Germany in the 1930s but common throughout Europe during the same period and even earlier in the USA (e.g. 63 000 Swedish people were sterilised between 1935 and 1976 – Jackson 2001, p. 45).

Right to reproduce

We have briefly looked at the idea of a 'right to reproduce' in relation to assisted conception (Chapter 9). The importance of the concept in this context was first noted in the case of *Re D.* (1976) when the court refused to allow an 11-year-old girl with Sotos syndrome to be sterilised (the syndrome is characterised by epilepsy, clumsiness, behavioural problems, aggression and impaired mental function). The main reason given by the judge was that sterilisation 'involved the deprivation of a basic human right, namely the right to reproduce, which, if performed for non-therapeutic reasons (i.e. to safeguard and promote the patient's way of life) and without her consent would be a violation of that right'.

Re D. prompted wide debate about the scope and meaning of the 'right to reproduce'. Was the 'right' an absolute one, for example, or did it mean (as was more widely believed) that you have a right to choose whether or not to reproduce (Mason 1998, p. 85)? Interpreted this way, if a patient is unable to give consent as a result of mental incapacity then there is no moral objection to the court assuming this right on the patient's behalf.

Best interests

Moral objections to non-consensual sterilisation tend to focus on the uncertainty and subjective nature of the concept of 'best interests'. It is the guiding principle justifying medical intervention in cases of incapacity and is widely used (see Chapter 11 for reform proposals). Yet because it is a subjective concept it invariably reflects the values and attitudes of those making the decisions. So what does it mean?

The first point to stress is that a decision that sterilisation is in the patient's best interests is not the same as saying that it is medically necessary (i.e. that it is therapeutic). Of course it may well be that that is the case – for example, when a hysterectomy is performed because a woman has cancer of the uterus. But in other situations a sterilisation may be carried out for social reasons. As such, it will be harder to justify on moral grounds. Sterilisations that are not medically necessary are often described as *non-therapeutic*. In other words they are performed to protect a patient's lifestyle and enable her to lead a life in keeping with her needs and capacities. The kinds of 'social' reasons that are typically given to justify non-therapeutic sterilisations of learning disabled women are:

- They cannot cope with the complexities of contraception
- Despite being sexually active they have no understanding of the relationship between sex and pregnancy
- The pain and emotional trauma of childbirth (or abortion) would be too great a burden
- Avoiding pregnancy frees them mentally from the constraints of their fertility and allows them to express their sexuality
- Lacking maternal instincts and unable to understand the responsibilities of parenthood, it is unlikely that such women could ever care for a child, yet they would be traumatised if their babies were taken away from them.

Reflective activity

Which of the above reasons do you think is a) morally most acceptable and b) least acceptable? Why?

Legal aspects

Over the last 30 years a number of cases have reached the courts concerning the non-consensual sterilisation of women, children and most recently men. Although decisions like these have inevitably to be made on a case-by-case basis a set of principles have emerged about the factors that all involved in the decision-making process are expected to consider. These are now incorporated in *Practice Note: Medical and Welfare Decisions for Adults who Lack Capacity* (2001) 2 FLR 158. The main points follow.

Court involvement

Before a person (either an adult or child) can be sterilised without their consent the court's permission must be obtained. This rule applies in virtually all cases of non-consensual sterilisation – the only exception being when they need to be performed for therapeutic as opposed to contraceptive purposes, i.e. they are medically necessary.

When will the court authorise a sterilisation?

The court will only allow a person to be sterilised if it is in his/her 'best interests'. In other words it must promote and safeguard his/her welfare. The concept of 'best interests' is very broad and so includes medical, emotional and other social issues. It is self-evident, too, that the best interests of a man are not the same as those of a woman – because of obvious biological differences.

Factors the court will consider

The factors the courts will consider in applying the best interests test include evidence that:

- The patient lacks capacity
- The operation is needed because there is a real need, i.e. the patient can become pregnant and either has had or is likely to have sexual intercourse
- The physical and psychological consequences of pregnancy and childbirth have been fully considered, focusing especially on the patient's ability to care for or have a fulfilling relationship with a child
- There has been full consideration of all possible medical and surgical techniques and ways of dealing with the patient's problems – such as whether lesser measures (e.g. an intrauterine contraceptive device) might be a better option.

Over to you

Read (and compare) the summary of the following cases on how the courts have interpreted the best interests test in Mason *et al.* 2002, pp. 123–135:

- *Re H.G.* (1993) – sterilisation authorised for 17-year-old with epilepsy
- *Re L.C.* (1997) – sterilisation refused as no real risk of pregnancy
- *Re S.* (2000) – permission given for IUD rather than hysterectomy
- *Re A.* (2000) – sterilisation refused for male with Down's syndrome.

Key points **Top tips**

- The Mental Capacity Bill 2004 introduces a statutory 'best interests' test (see Chapter 11) – if the bill becomes law, the 2001 Practice Note will no longer apply

Key points Top tips

- The court's prior approval will almost always be required when patients lack capacity to consent to sterilisation
- The guiding principle in non-consensual sterilisation is the patient's 'best interests'

Legality of family planning methods

Birth control

In this section we briefly consider the legality of various methods of birth control.

Contraception

There is no legal definition of contraception but it is nevertheless assumed that it covers any birth control method that prevents fertilisation. It therefore includes barrier methods such as the condom and diaphragm as well as oral and long-acting contraceptives. Other than ensuring that valid legal consent is given (see Chapter 6) none of these methods presents any legal difficulties. However, if a health professional were to prescribe oral or injectable contraceptives without taking a full history (medical, family or menstrual), or conducting any appropriate tests or examinations then the health professional could face a negligence claim (see Chapter 5).

Postcoital methods

Postcoital birth control – the 'morning-after pill' and intrauterine contraceptive devices (IUDs) – are designed to work after the embryo has formed (i.e. after fertilisation but before implantation). This explains why they cannot be accurately described as contraception – which prevents fertilisation. Although generally these methods of birth control are unproblematic, in some cases it can be important to distinguish between them. Thus the morning-after pill is normally prescribed within 72 hours of unprotected sex. As such it does prevent implantation (as does an IUD fitted before intercourse). But legal problems can arise if an IUD is fitted postcoitally – because then (depending on precisely when intercourse took place and when the device was fitted) it could dislodge an embryo that has already implanted. In such cases compliance with the Abortion Act 1967 is necessary.

Abortifacients

The distinction between abortion and contraception is further complicated by techniques such as so-called 'abortion pills' (mifepristone, commonly known as RU486). The problem is that these techniques can make it difficult to tell whether a pregnancy is being prevented or terminated. If used to prevent implantation they are like any other pre-implantation postcoital method of birth control. On the other hand, if used to dislodge an implanted fertilised egg from the lining of the uterus they amount to an abortion – and so again must comply with the Abortion Act 1967.

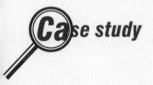

Case study

Susan's unwanted baby – damages for 'wrongful' birth

Susan is 39 and has three children under 10. Her husband James has recently been diagnosed with a progressive neurological condition. Although he can still work it is very unlikely that he will be able to so for very much longer. They therefore decide that Susan should be sterilised. Several months after the operation Susan is very surprised to discover that she is pregnant. Refusing an abortion, she has just given birth to a healthy baby girl (Diana). Desperately anxious about how she is gong to cope – James is now in a wheelchair and unable to work at all – Susan wants to claim damages for the 'wrongful' birth of Diana.

Reflective activity

1. Can Susan recover damages for the unplanned birth of Diana?
2. What are the moral implications of such a claim?

Case study continued

1. Damages for the unwanted birth of Diana

Susan's claim for damages (which is usually called a 'wrongful birth' action) can be broken down into several elements – for pregnancy-related expenses, for the pain and suffering caused by childbirth and for the costs of bringing up a child. Compensation for the first two heads of claims – pregnancy expenses (such as loss of earnings) and the pain, etc. of childbirth itself – have long been recognised by the courts. Much more controversial has been the claim for the costs of raising a normal, healthy child. Until recently these too were recognised by the courts, albeit reluctantly. But the latest case on this aspect of a claim arising from a failed sterilisation – *McFarlane* v. *Tayside Health Board* (1999) – has made it clear that the costs of rearing a healthy child are not recoverable.

2. Moral implications of 'unwanted baby' claims

The reasons why the courts have decided to reject compensating parents for the cost of their unplanned child's upbringing are threefold:

- The cost to health authorities would not be proportionate to the doctor's actual negligence – in other words, damages for a child's upbringing would be far greater than the degree of negligence that led to the child's birth
- It would be 'unseemly and contrary to public morality' to compensate parents for the birth of a healthy child
- It is unfair, unreasonable and unjust to use scarce NHS resources to compensate parents for the cost of having a healthy child.

Reflective activity

Do you agree that it is unjust to compensate parents for the birth of a healthy child? If not, why not?

Top tips

Wrongful birth actions may be available in the following circumstances:

- Failure to detect foetal abnormality
- Giving a pregnant woman incorrect information about the results of a prenatal test
- Assisted conception (if a disabled child is born as a result of inadequate screening of donor gametes)

The relationship between law and ethics

Similarities between law and ethics

- **Status of the foetus**. Law and ethics ask the same questions – does the foetus have legal and moral status and, if so, what kind of protection should it be entitled to?
- **Abortion**.
  - The Abortion Act 1967 recognises the legal and moral status of the foetus by, for example, limiting 'late' abortions
  - The Abortion Act 1967 attempts to balance the legal and moral rights of the foetus and the pregnant woman
  - The 'conscience' clause in the Abortion Act acknowledges the moral and legal rights of third parties to refuse to participate in abortions.
- **Non-consensual sterilisation**.
  - The idea that there is a 'right to reproduce' is recognised in both law and ethics but neither regards it as an absolute right
  - In deciding whether to sterilise a person without their consent, law and ethics adopt the same guiding principle – the 'best interests' test.

Differences between law and ethics

- **Status of the foetus**. The foetus is not a legal person but does acquire legal rights *in utero* that crystallise at birth; in contrast, many claim that the foetus's moral status is established well before (e.g. at conception or when it becomes a 'person').
- **Abortion**. Denying that the foetus has any legal status (and thus no legal right to life) means that its moral claims are of little practical significance.
- **Non-consensual sterilisation**. The court's involvement in almost all sterilisation cases reflects the law's strong commitment to promoting the patient's 'best interests' rather than the interests or convenience of carers or the public; the ethical basis of the 'best interests' test is weaker, or at least less well articulated.

RRRR*Rapid recap*

Check your progress so far by working through each of the following questions.

1. Is the foetus a legal person?
2. What is meant by the claim that 'the foetus has a right to life'?
3. When is an abortion legal?
4. What is a 'wrongful birth' claim?

If you have difficulty with more than one of the questions, read through the section again to refresh your understanding before moving on.

References

Dimond, B. (2002) *Legal Aspects of Midwifery*, 2nd edn. Books for Midwives, Edinburgh.

Glover, J. (1990) *Causing Death and Saving Lives*. Penguin, Harmondsworth.

Harris, J. (1985) *The Value of Life: An introduction to medical ethics*. Routledge, London.

Jackson, E. (2001) *Regulating Reproduction: Law, technology and autonomy*. Hart, Oxford.

McDonagh, E. (2002) Models of motherhood in the abortion debate: self-sacrifice versus self-defence. In: *Ethical Issues in Maternal–Foetal Medicine* (ed. D.L. Dickenson). Cambridge University Press, Cambridge.

Mason, J.K. (1998) *Medico-legal Aspects of Reproduction and Parenthood*, 2nd edn. Dartmouth, Aldershot.

Mason, J.K., McCall Smith, R.A. and Laurie, G.T. (2002) *Law and Medical Ethics*, 6th edn. Butterworths, London.

Thomson, J.J. (1971) A defense of abortion. Philosophy and Public Affairs, Princeton University Press. Reprinted in: *Applied Ethics* (ed. P. Singer). Oxford University Press, Oxford.

Tooley, M. (1983) *Abortion and Infanticide*. Oxford University Press, Oxford.

Tschudin V. (2003) *Ethics in nursing: the caring relationship*, 3rd edn. Butterworth Heinemann, Edinburgh.

Warren, M.A. (1993) Abortion. In: *A Companion to Ethics* (ed. P. Singer). Blackwell, Oxford.

Warren, M.A. (1997) On the moral and legal status of abortion. In: *Ethics in Practice* (ed. H. LaFollette). Blackwell, Oxford.

Whyte, A. (1997) Fertile ground. *Nursing Times* **93**(14) 16.

Caring for people with mental health problems and/ or learning disabilities

Learning outcomes

By the end of this chapter you should be able to:

- Discuss the moral and legal implications of compulsory detention and treatment
- Describe the key provisions of the Mental Health Act 1983
- Understand how health-care decisions are made for those with learning disabilities.

Introduction

It is currently estimated that on average one person in four in the UK will experience some kind of mental health problem in the course of a year. And, although psychotic illnesses are rare (affecting about 1% of the population), depression alone will affect one in six people at some point in their life (Mental Health Foundation 2003). Given these statistics it is no exaggeration to say that mental illness is a huge social problem. Of course, different mental health problems affect people differently – ranging from worries we all may experience as part of our everyday lives to suicidal depression. Yet mental illness can profoundly affect some people's lives. Under the Mental Health Act 1983, for example, people can be compulsorily detained in hospital and treated against their will (sometimes for months, if not years).

That these draconian powers need to be justified – both morally and legally – is therefore self-evident. Legally the concern must be to make sure that people are only deprived of their liberty if stringent legal procedures (in the Mental Health Act 1983) have been followed. These are therefore described in some detail in this chapter. Proposed reforms to the current law are also briefly discussed (although these are not expected to come into effect until 2006 at the earliest).

As to the moral issues, these focus mainly on the conflict between autonomy and paternalism, i.e. in what circumstances it is morally acceptable to limit an individual's right to run his/her own life by making decisions on his/her behalf? We then discuss how decisions about medical treatment are made on behalf of people with learning disabilities. The chapter ends with an outline of the ethical and legal issues raised by research involving adults who are incompetent.

As in other chapters, we begin by defining some key terms.

What is a mental health problem?

The term 'mental health problem' covers a very wide spectrum but the six most common types of problem are severe depression, panic attacks, schizophrenia, dementia, eating disorders and alcohol and drug addiction (Mental Health Foundation 2003). Although this 'list' may not be controversial there are several difficulties with the term 'mental health problem'. The following points illustrate some of them.

- 'Mental illness' (the term used in this chapter) is commonly used in the literature to describe people with mental disorders and other mental health problems; in other words these labels are used very broadly (and often inaccurately).

- There is no universally agreed cut-off point between 'normal' behaviour and that described as 'mental illness'. What is considered abnormal behaviour or an abnormal reaction to circumstances differs between cultures as well as between social groups within the same culture.

- Use of terms such as 'mental illness' and 'mental disorder' can be misleading, as they imply that all mental health problems are caused solely by medical or biological factors. In fact, most result from a complex interaction of biological, social and personal factors.

- The so-called 'antipsychiatry' movement – prominent in the 1960s and associated with, for example, Szasz (1970) – claims that there is no such thing as mental illness. Rather it is a term applied to people who behave in a way that society finds unacceptable – they may, for example, have an eccentric life style, hold bizarre beliefs or be 'antisocial'. In other words, our attitudes to mental illness are shaped by our value judgements – about what we think are desirable or acceptable standards of behaviour (Hendrick 2000, p. 174).

> ### Over to you
>
> Read Bartlett and Sandland 2003, ch. 1. Consider how they define and describe attitudes to 'the insane'.

Why is a diagnosis of a mental illness important?

A diagnosis of mental illness is important because of the huge impact it can have on a person's life. These include the following.

Stigma

Although we may no longer treat people with mental illness as we did in Victorian times, general ignorance about it means that it still attracts a lot of stigma. The media, for example, typically (albeit misleadingly) portray the mentally ill as a lurking (but hidden) menace in society who are not only poor and homeless but also violent. Alternatively, and just as misleadingly, the 'insane' are romanticised as mad artistic geniuses. Either way, although statistically the mad killer (or genius) is rare, these images encourage people to think of the mentally ill as an entirely separate category from 'people like us'. Given these images it is not surprising that people with mental illness attract fear, hostility and disapproval rather than compassion, support and understanding.

Discrimination

Because of our society's prejudiced attitude towards the mentally ill they are routinely discriminated against – in the workplace, housing, leisure, social and health services. And this discrimination is likely to last a long time. This is because, once someone has been labelled or stereotyped as mentally ill, there is almost nothing they can do to shed the stigma (personal, legal and social) that the label carries. Thus, even though, as Chadwick and Tadd point out (1992, p. 34), labelling people is commonplace (and can be harmless), categorising people as 'mentally ill' means that society comes to expect and indeed looks for instances of behaviour that justify the label.

Compulsory intervention

A finding of mental illness, in law, can result in a person not only being compulsorily detained in hospital (for months, if not years) but also losing control over their property and affairs. Furthermore, they may be treated without their consent – sometimes with powerful chemicals or electricity.

Key points | **Top tips**

- For details of a national anti-discrimination campaign aimed at tackling the stigma and discrimination faced by people with mental health problems, visit www.nimhe.org.uk/priorities.mhpromotion

- The term 'mental health problem' is very broad and can cover a range of different disorders
- A diagnosis of mental disorder or illness can profoundly affect a person's life – resulting in discrimination and compulsory detention and treatment

Is compulsory intervention morally acceptable?

As we have seen above, a diagnosis of mental illness can have very serious repercussions, especially if it results in a person being admitted, detained and treated in hospital against his/her will. So what moral justification is there for restricting the liberty of people with mental illness? One is to protect the public and the other is to protect the mentally ill from themselves.

The protection of others

Justifying compulsory intervention on the basis that society needs protection strongly suggests that people with a psychiatric illness are a threat to the community. In some cases, albeit rarely, this may be true because they have committed a serious crime. However, in the vast majority of cases it is because of the fear that they may do so unless they are detained in hospital and/or compulsorily treated.

Yet fear (on its own) can only be a sufficiently strong moral ground to deprive someone of their liberty if we have a very clear idea of what that person might do. In other words, we can only justify compulsory intervention in the lives of those who are mentally ill if they really are 'dangerous', i.e. are likely to harm other people.

The problem here is, of course, that terms like 'dangerous' (and 'harm') are very difficult to define objectively. Nor is it generally possible to accurately predict who might become dangerous. This means that, although we might all agree that society has a right to protect itself from dangerous or harmful conduct (i.e. that which the law defines as criminal), we are less likely to agree on what other kind of other harm it has the right to protect itself against.

The protection of self

The other justification for compulsory interference in the lives of the mentally ill is that it is in their best interests. In short, paternalistic intervention is necessary to stop them harming themselves, i.e. their physical (and mental) health will otherwise suffer.

The major problem with this justification is the need to show why people who are mentally ill should be subject to compulsory action for their own good when we let other people – smokers, heavy drinkers, sky divers and so on – act as they please regardless of the danger they put themselves in. The usual reply to this kind of argument is that the mentally ill lack the ability to make rational choices.

Thus, even though few philosophers can agree on what it means to make a rational decision, most accept that some people – at least those with severely irrational beliefs – are more likely to harm themselves and act in ways that are not in their best interests. As Lindley notes (1978, p. 42), a man who thinks he is Superman (and so can fly) can justifiably be stopped from jumping off a cliff. On the other hand, it is far harder to justify preventing people who have the capacity to reason (and make decisions) from smoking or drinking. This is because, once they have been informed about and understand the risks they are exposing themselves to, it is up to them to decide whether or not to smoke or drink themselves to an early death.

Reflective activity

Do you agree that society has a right to protect itself from 'dangerous people'? If so, how would you define 'dangerous'?

Key points | Top tips

- The moral justification for compulsory intervention twofold, i.e. a) to protect the public and b) to protect the mentally ill for themselves

The Mental Health Act 1983

In this section we focus on some of the key aspects of the Mental Health Act 1983 (the MHA). These include:

- Informal admission (of 'voluntary' patients)
- Compulsory admission
- Compulsory treatment
- Nurses' roles
- Patients' rights.

You need to be aware, however, that the MHA covers many other areas – e.g. the activities of the Court of Protection, which manages the financial affairs and property of people who are mentally disordered.

We start with some introductory information:

- The MHA only applies to a person with a '**mental disorder**'
- All the terms are further defined in the MHA (section 1) except 'mental illness', which guidelines suggests means either sustained cognitive impairment or, essentially, psychosis (i.e. delusions, hallucinations, disordered thinking)
- Although mental illness is defined very broadly in the MHA (and so can include people with mental handicaps and adults with brain damage), the Act also makes it clear that people cannot be regarded, in law, as mentally disordered because they are dependent on drugs or alcohol, promiscuous or sexually deviant
- The MHA is concerned only with treatment (or assessment) of the mental disorder) and not with treatment of an unrelated physical disorder
- The MHA is supplemented by a code of practice (the latest edition was issued in 1999). The code gives guidance to practitioners by explaining the law and how it should be interpreted. Although it sets standards of 'good practice' it does not strictly have legal force.

Informal admission (section 131) – 'voluntary' patients

Admission for treatment on an informal basis accounts for the vast majority of people received into psychiatric care. Because they are admitted without the use of compulsory powers they are often called 'voluntary patients'. Overall, section 131 of the MHA encourages admission without any legal formality (similar, in other words, to the way in which patients enter hospital for physical disorders). The legal status of informal patients is very different from those detained compulsorily because, in theory at least, they can go (and come) as they please, i.e. leave when they want to go, and reject treatment (if they are competent). As we shall see, however, they too can be detained against their will.

Compulsory admission – when is it lawful to detain people against their will?

The main sections under which patients can be admitted and detained against their will are summarised in the box below.

Keywords

Mental disorder
Mental illness, arrested or incomplete development of mind, psychopathic disorder and any other disorder or disability of mind (section 1, MHA 1983); the term 'mental disorder' is a therefore a collective term (with five subdivisions)

Summary of powers to admit and detain patients

Assessment order (section 2)

This order allows compulsory admission and detention for up to 28 days. It is a short-term measure that applies to all five forms of disorder and is designed for a very specific purpose, namely an assessment of the patient's condition. Detention can only be lawful if several conditions are met. Two doctors must 'recommend' detention and the order must be applied for by the 'nearest relative' (NR) or an 'approved social worker' (ASW).

Treatment order (section 3)

This long-term provision can last initially up to 6 months and on first renewal for a further 6 months. Subsequent renewals can last for a year at a time. It applies to patients suffering from mental illness, psychopathic disorder, mental impairment and severe mental impairment. The order is made by the NR, or by an ASW (if the NR does not object) on the recommendation of two doctors.

Emergency order (section 4)

This order lasts up to 72 hours. It applies to all forms of disorder. It is made by an ASW or NR but only needs the recommendation of one doctor. The intention behind the order is that it should only be used only for 'genuine' emergencies. It is typically used as a short-cut variant of ordinary admission, to which it can later be converted.

Voluntary patients (section 5(2))

This power lasts up to 72 hours. It applies to voluntary patients (with all forms of disorder) as well as those who are in hospital but are not being treated for a mental disorder, whom the doctor thinks 'ought' to be detained. The effect of the order is that the informal patient's voluntary status is converted to that of compulsory detention. Detention is short-term but is usually, although not inevitably, the first step to more long-term compulsory detention.

Voluntary patients (section 5(4))

Prescribed nurses (i.e. those qualified in mental disorder) have 'holding' powers of 6 hours. This allows them to detain an informal patient (suffering from any of the five disorders) who wants to leave hospital. Stricter tests than apply to doctors must be met before the power can be used – immediate restraint must be necessary.

Notes

- The legal definition of a 'nearest relative' is complex. It includes husbands and wives, unmarried couples, children and so on (section 26).
- Other routes into compulsory detention include:
  - Section 135, which gives the police authority to enter a person's home if it is felt that person is a danger to themselves or others as a result of a mental disorder
  - Section 136, which gives the police various powers to remove mentally disordered people from public places.
- Irrespective of how patients get to be compulsorily detained, the process is usually called 'sectioning'.

Reflective activity

What does the fact that 'minority groups' are statistically over-represented in the detention statistics imply about attitudes to (and the definition of) mental illness?

Statistics reveal that 24 000 people were sectioned in England in 2002/03, compared to 19 000 in 1992/93. What does this increase suggest about the success of the current mental health system?

Top tips

- 90% of the 250 000 people admitted to psychiatric care each year (in England and Wales) arrive 'informally' under section 131
- To find out more about mental health statistics visit the Mental Health Foundation website at www.mentalhealth.org.uk (it is the biggest, most comprehensive website on mental health in the UK)

Compulsory treatment

Ethical issues

The moral justification for depriving patients of their rights to consent to or reject treatment is twofold: first, even if some patients are not morally responsible for their behaviour, society is entitled to protect itself from conduct that threatens its safety. Secondly, compulsory treatment may be justified on the basis of the patient's own interests, i.e. to protect him/her from self-harm.

Underlying these moral justifications is, of course, the assumption that treatment will, if not cure the patient, then at the very least help him/her in some way. But is this so? Anti-psychiatrists, such as Szasz (1970), would almost certainly disagree, claiming that patients labelled mentally ill end up being imprisoned in institutions, which can only do damage by making it much less likely that they can be socially and psychologically rehabilitated.

It is also important to question the moral basis for compulsory treatment because without such an enquiry patients may be denied the right to make a whole range of decisions (extending well beyond treatment). In other words there is a real risk that their competence will not be thoroughly assessed – once they have been labelled 'mentally ill' they are simply assumed to be incapable.

Legal provisions

Part IV of the Mental Health Act 1983 contains several provisions authorising compulsory treatment for mental disorder. They apply to most detained patients (i.e. those detained under sections 2 and 3, but not, for example, under the emergency section 4 order, the section 5 holding powers or sections 135 and 136). Exceptionally, section 57 also applies to informal patients. Part IV (which is very complex) is summarised in the box below.

Summary of treatment provisions in the Mental Health Act 1983

Psychosurgery and surgical implants (section 57)

Treatments regulated by section 57 are the most drastic and intrusive. Psychosurgery is defined as any surgery that destroys brain tissue or functioning. The section also covers surgical implants to reduce male sex drive. Both these treatments can only be carried out with the patient's consent (which must be verified by three independent people). There must also be a second opinion supporting it, i.e. one of the three (a doctor) must also certify in writing (following consultation with two others, one of whom must be a nurse) that the treatment should be given. This section applies to informal patients.

Electroconvulsive therapy and long-term drug treatment (section 58)

Opinions about the use of electroconvulsive therapy (ECT) are very divided – in particular about its long-term benefits. It is now used mainly for depressive disorders and affective psychoses. Long-term medication – psychiatric drugs (which constitute around one-quarter of all prescriptions dispensed by the NHS) – includes antipsychotics, antidepressants and anti-anxiety drugs. They are long term if they are given to patients for longer than 3 months from the time the patient was first given drugs – drugs given before then are regulated by section 63 (see below). These treatments are only lawful if either a) the patient consents or b) there has been a second opinion, i.e. an independent doctor has approved of them being carried out (following consultation with two others, one of whom must be a nurse). In other words, the second opinion is an alternative to the patient's consent.

All other forms of treatment (including medication; section 63)

This section allows medical treatment (apart from that covered by sections 57 and 58) to be given without consent to detained patients for the mental disorder for which they are suffering. Because the courts have interpreted section 63 very broadly it seems that non-psychiatric care can be given without consent in a wide range of circumstances – provided that the physical problems are related to the mental disorder, either in their origins or their effects.

Urgent treatment (section 62)

In certain circumstances, section 62 allows treatment to be carried out without the need to comply with the various legal safeguards of sections 57 and 58. Basically,

continued

section 62 is limited to treatment that is immediately and minimally necessary. In practice it tends to be used when a patient needs drug treatment that would otherwise be caught by the 3-month rule.

Notes

- The term 'medical treatment' in Part IV is very broadly interpreted. It includes nursing as well as 'care, habilation and rehabilitation under medical supervision'. In short, it covers physical treatment, medication and psychotherapy, i.e. anything designed to treat, control or manage the patient (including seclusion and restraint).

- Medical treatment must be given for the patient's mental disorder. In other words, the Act does not authorise treatment for physical disorders that are unrelated to the patient's mental disorder.

Key points ~~Top tips~~

- Part IV of the Mental Health Act 1983 authorises the compulsory treatment of detained patients in hospital

Nurses' role under the Mental Health Act 1983

Applications for detention are normally made by nearest relatives or approved social workers (but note a nurse's 6-hour holding power under section 5(4) – see the box on page 193). You may nevertheless be involved in the care of patients in several other ways. For example:

- If consulted about whether a long-term section 3 treatment order should be renewed
- Making sure that paperwork is correct
- Providing information to patients, e.g. about why they are being detained and the effects of detention
- Informing patients about their rights, e.g. to apply to a Mental Health Review Tribunal (see below)
- Explaining the rules relating to consent to treatment and the role of the Mental Health Act Commission (see below).

Compulsory treatment in the community

The focus of the MHA is on hospital treatment. However, in the last 20 years or so there has been a move towards treatment in the community. While guardianship orders (sections 7–10 of the MHA) give guardians several powers – e.g. to require a patient to attend (at places and times) for medical treatment – there are no means of enforcing them. Nor are they effective in preventing so-called 'revolving door admissions'. These arise when patients have a chronic condition (e.g. schizophrenia) that is well controlled by drugs. However, if they stop the medication (after being discharged) they may relapse and then need compulsory treatment in hospital. And once they are again discharged the cycle is repeated (Hope *et al.* 2003, p. 151).

To fill in the gaps in the legislation the Mental Health (Patients in the Community) Act 1995 was passed. This added several sections to the MHA (sections 25A–25J). The intention was to ensure that patients obtained the aftercare services specified in the MHA, known as 'supervised discharge'. Although the 1995 Act gives more powers to guardians – e.g. the power to take patients who are over 16 (using force if necessary) to a place to receive treatment – it stops short of authorising compulsory treatment in the community (Dimond 2002, pp. 413–414).

Key points **Top tips**

- For details of care, control and services in the community for mentally disordered people, read Bartlett and Sandland 2003, ch. 9

Patients' rights under the Mental Health Act 1983

The MHA gives detained patients several important rights. Here are some of the most important:

- **To leave hospital**. There are several options here: patients can, for example, challenge their detention by applying to a Mental Health Review Tribunal for discharge, or they can make an informal application to the managers of the hospital (Montgomery 2003, pp. 338–342).

- **To information**. Patients have the right to the information specified in section 132 – i.e. under what sections they are detained (and their effect); their rights to apply to a Mental Health Review Tribunal; the MHA's discharge provisions and those about compulsory treatment; the effect of the code of practice and the powers of the Mental Health Act Commission.

- **Access to a Mental Health Review Tribunal**. These are independent bodies whose basic function is to safeguard the rights of detained patients and make sure their detention is regularly reviewed; basically their role is to decide whether a patient should continue to be detained.

- **Access to the Mental Health Act Commission**. The Commission has several protective and supervisory functions, including visiting and hearing complaints from detained patients, and reviewing treatment (under sections 57 and 58).

- **To services**. Certain patients, most notably those detained for treatment or following criminal proceedings, have a legal right to 'aftercare' when they leave hospital (see section 117).

The future – reform of the Mental Health Act 1983

Mental health law is currently under review. Following a long period of consultation, the government published a draft mental health bill in 2002. It was widely criticised, prompting fears that, because of the way mental disorder was defined, a far wider group of people would be brought under compulsion than under current legislation. Even more controversial were several new provisions authorising:

- The compulsory treatment of patients in the community (defined very broadly to include prisons)

- The detention of people with severe personality disorders – even though they had not committed any crime.

Undoubtedly, these new powers reflected the government's preoccupation with the danger posed by people with psychiatric illness. However, critics (which included the Royal College of Psychiatrists) argued that they would not only violate patients' basic human rights but were also unnecessary – because the vast majority of mentally ill people are simply not dangerous. In fact, the number of people killed by the mentally ill has been steadily falling since the 1970s (Bartlett and Sandland 2003, p. 3).

Lack of support for the bill prompted the government to revise its plans and a second draft is expected in the near future. It is unlikely, however, that a new mental health Act will be on the statute books before 2006/07 at the earliest.

Top tips

- For up-to-date information about proposals for reform, see www.doh.gov.uk/mentalhealth

Caring for people with learning disabilities

In this section we look at the principles governing the care and treatment of patients with learning disabilities who lack the ability to make their own decisions (i.e. they are incompetent). These principles also cover patients compulsorily detained in hospital (under the Mental Health Act 1983) and informal patients who need treatment for physical illnesses or conditions that are not related to their mental disorders (see the box below).

Jonathan's appendicitis

Jonathan is very depressed and has been detained under section 3 of the MHA for the last 6 months. He has recently been complaining of stomach pains and has been sick, with a high temperature. Jonathan is diagnosed with appendicitis and an immediate operation is recommended. Jonathan refuses his consent for the operation.

This situation is not covered by the MHA but Jonathan could be forced to have the surgery against his will under the common law principle of 'best interests'. In other words, he could be treated without consent. For this to be lawful, of course, he would have to be incompetent, i.e. lack capacity.

Notes

- If Jonathan has learning disabilities he could similarly be treated without his consent (under the 'best interests' principle) – providing, of course, that he was incompetent
- Treatment under the 'best interests' principle would also be lawful if Jonathan was in hospital as an informal patient (and incompetent).

Ethical issues

It is not difficult to justify treating patients without their consent if they lack autonomy – because of temporary or permanent incapacity – on the basis of paternalism (Chapter 6), especially if treatment is necessary to save their lives. It is, however, less easy to do so when their lives are not threatened or when treatment is controversial (as, for example, in sterilisation cases; Chapter 10). Questions then need to be asked about who should make medical decisions for them and on what basis.

As we shall see, the law authorises non-consensual treatment if it is in the patient's best interests. The best interests approach is also morally acceptable – providing, of course, that you do not simply assume that just because someone has a learning disability s/he is incompetent. In short, you should do all you can to respect the autonomy of patients with learning disabilities and promote their independence whenever possible (UKCC 1998).

> ### Over to you
>
> Read UKCC 1998 for guidance on other issues relating to the care of people with learning disabilities.

Legal issues – when is (and what) treatment is lawful?

How can you be sure that proposed care or treatment is within the law? According to *Re F.* (1990), the treatment of incapacitated adult patients at common law is lawful provided the following conditions are met:

- Adult patients who lack capacity can be treated without their consent providing 'treatment' is in their best interests
- Treatment is in a patient's best interests if it is carried out either to save his/her life, to improve his/her physical or mental health or to prevent it from deteriorating
- The word 'treatment' is broadly interpreted and so includes minor routine procedures as well as major surgery; it also covers other types of care such as washing, bathing and so on
- In interpreting the term 'best interests' health professionals must follow 'a responsible body of professional practice' (Chapter 5).

One of the main problems with the best interests test is that it gives health professionals a very wide discretion to decide in what circumstances treatment should be given. But this will change if proposals in the draft Mental Capacity Bill (2004) come into force. The bill introduces new decision making mechanisms to allow welfare and health-care decisions to be taken on behalf of persons lacking capacity. One of its key reforms is to formalise the best interests test – by, for example, specifying a checklist of factors that decision-makers must consider. These are:

- Whether the person is likely to regain capacity in the future
- The need to include the person as far as possible in decision-making
- The past and present wishes of the person concerned
- The views of other people concerned with the person who lacks capacity.

Key points Top tips

- The treatment of incompetent patients (with physical disorders) is governed by the 'best interests' test

Research

Ethical issues

In this section we briefly consider the ethical issues raised by research with vulnerable adults, i.e. those with mental health problems or learning disabilities. It is widely recognised that research with such groups is particularly problematic, i.e. they are more vulnerable than other people to discrimination and exploitation (Royal College of Nursing 2003). For example, researchers may be tempted to assume that, because incapacitated adults are receiving treatment without their consent – even perhaps against their expressed wishes – it must be morally acceptable to combine that treatment with research. To ensure that this does not happen, most ethical guidance, while not prohibiting therapeutic research on incompetent adults altogether, nevertheless recommends that very strict safeguards are put in place (Chalmers and Lindley 2001).

What is more problematic is whether non-therapeutic research is also ethical. Given that there is no direct benefit to the participant, this kind of research is harder to justify. Nevertheless current guidance (e.g. Medical Research Council 2001) does permit it, providing, of course, that several stringent conditions are met. For example, the risks involved should not be greater than those encountered in everyday life or during routine physical or psychological tests (Hope *et al.* 2003, p. 201).

Legal issues

Research involving incompetent adults is problematic because English law does not currently authorise a proxy system whereby consent can be given on their behalf. This raises the question as to when, if at all, incompetent adults can be volunteered for research. As yet, no English court has had to decide this specific point. Nonetheless, most legal texts assume that, providing the research is therapeutic, incompetent adults can be involved. It is only lawful, however, if it is in their best interests. In contrast, the legality of non-therapeutic research is more doubtful. This explains why most legal commentators recommend that the court's permission be sought before it is undertaken.

Key points | **Top tips**

Be aware:

- That the draft Mental Capacity Bill 2004 supports therapeutic research on incompetent adults
- Of the impact of EU Directive 2001/20/EC (which may limit therapeutic research on incapacitated adults)

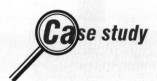 **Case study**

Penny's anorexia nervosa – can she be force fed?

Penny is 21 and suffers from anorexia. Life has not been kind to her. Her mother died when she was 7 and her father, who was successfully caring for her, was killed in a freak accident a few years later. She lived in several foster homes but all the placements broke down for one reason or another. At her last home she was sexually abused by her foster brother. She ran away and became a drug addict. Several weeks ago Penny took an overdose. She has since refused to eat and her weight is now dangerously low. There is little doubt that if she continues to refuse to eat her health and possibly her life will be in danger. A decision is made that she should be 'sectioned' under the Mental Health Act 1983 and force-fed.

Reflective activity

Is force-feeding lawful under the MHA?

Case study continued

The short answer is yes, providing the conditions in the MHA (section 63) are met. These are:

- That the patient is detained under the Act (e.g. under section 3)
- That what is proposed must count as 'medical treatment' and
- That the treatment (i.e. force-feeding) must constitute treatment for the mental disorder from which the patient is suffering.

All these conditions have been interpreted in a series of cases in the 1990s. From this it is now clear:

- That 'sectioning' of patients with anorexia nervosa is lawful, i.e. it is recognised as a mental disorder under the MHA (*Riverside Health NHS Trust v. Fox* [1994])
- That the phrase 'medical treatment' is interpreted very widely as a 'range of acts ancillary to core treatment'. As such it extends to force-feeding (*B. v. Croydon HA* [1995])
- That feeding by nasogastric tube does constitute treatment for the mental disorder of anorexia nervosa (*Re K.B.* [1994]). The problem dealt with in *Re K.B.* was whether force-feeding was given as treatment for the mental disorder or for the patient's physical symptoms – i.e. to increase weight. The judge accepted the argument that the patient was suffering from an eating disorder and that relieving symptoms was just as much part of treatment as relieving the underlying cause.

To summarise, it is clear then that Penny can be treated (i.e. force-fed) under section 63 of the MHA regardless of her competence. Note too that she can also be fed by force under the common law 'best interests' principle (if she lacks capacity).

Reflective activity

Do you think force-feeding Penny is morally right? Give reasons.

The relationship between law and ethics

Similarities between law and ethics

- The legal and ethical principles justifying compulsory detention and treatment are broadly similar – protecting society and protecting patients from self-harm (i.e. from themselves).
- Compulsory detention and treatment is legally and ethically justified providing it properly balances the needs of the community with the rights of patients.
- The legal and ethical justification for treating incompetent patients is the 'best interests' principle.

Differences between law and ethics

- The MHA imposes strict conditions that must be complied with before patients can be compulsorily detained and treated; in contrast the ethical principles underpinning paternalistic intervention are less clearly expressed.
- The ethical and legal approach to the treatment of people with mental handicap or learning disability may be based on the same principle, i.e. the best interest test, but the legal test gives decision-makers less discretion to make a value judgement.

RRRR**Rapid recap**

Check your progress so far by working through each of the following questions.

1. How can you justify the compulsory detention and treatment of patients with mental disorders?
2. What does 'sectioning' mean?
3. What does the phrase 'informal admission' mean?
4. Can patients be force-fed?
5. When is treatment of patients with learning disabilities lawful?

If you have difficulty with more than one of the questions, read through the section again to refresh your understanding before moving on.

References

Bartlett, P. and Sandland, R. (2003) *Mental Health Law*. Blackstone Press, London.

Chadwick, R. and Tadd, W. (1992) *Ethics and Nursing Practice: A case study approach*. Macmillan, Basingstoke.

Chalmers, I. and Lindley, R.I. (2001) Double standards on informed consent to treatment. In: *Informed Consent in Medical Research* (eds L. Doyle and J. Tobias). BMJ Books, London.

Department of Health (1999) *Mental Health Act 1983: Code of practice*, 3rd edn. HMSO, London.

Dimond, B. (2002) *Legal Aspects of Nursing*, 3rd edn. Pearson Education, Harlow.

Hendrick, J. (2000) *Law and Ethics in Nursing and Health Care*. Stanley Thornes, Cheltenham.

Hope, T., Savulescu, J. and Hendrick, J. (2003) *Medical Ethics and Law: The core curriculum*. Churchill Livingstone, Edinburgh.

Lindley, R. (1978) Social philosophy. In: *What Philosophy Does* (R. Lindley, R. Fellows and G. Macdonald). Open Books, London.

Medical Research Council (2001) *Personal Information in Medical Research*. MRC Ethics Series. Medical Research Council, London.

Mental Health Foundation (2003) *Introduction to Mental Health*. Mental Health Foundation, London.

Montgomery, J. (2003) *Health Care Law*. Oxford University Press, Oxford.

Royal College of Nursing (2003) *Research Ethics*. Royal College of Nursing, London.

Szasz, T. (1970) *Ideology and Insanity: Essays on the psychiatric dehumanisation of man*. Doubleday, Garden City, NY.

UKCC (1998) *Guidelines for Mental Health and Learning Disabilities*. United Kingdom Central Council for Nursing, Midwifery and Health Visiting, London.

12

Caring for children and young people

Learning outcomes

By the end of this chapter you should be able to:

- Discuss the concept of childhood
- Consider the different approaches to the notion of children's rights
- Understand the legal and ethical framework governing consent, research and confidentiality
- Describe how the child protection system works.

Introduction

The care of children and adolescents (i.e. anyone under the age of 18) is governed by the same principles and professional standards discussed in previous chapters. Yet sometimes it may be legally and morally appropriate to classify them as special subjects. By special we mean that they may lack the physical and mental maturity to make their own decisions. If so, it is necessary for someone else to take them on their behalf.

But who has this power and in what circumstances can they exercise it? These are the kinds of question we consider in this chapter. Consequently, we focus on consent, research and confidentiality – all of which raise fundamental issues about the autonomy of patients under 18.

However, as we shall see, the fact that the law now requires you to give much greater weight than in the past to the views of children and adolescents can lead to some very poignant dilemmas in practice. The idea that children should have rights to make their own decisions is, however, a relatively modern one. And as we shall see below, it is one that very much reflects the type of childhood children now experience.

But what do we mean when we talk about childhood and children's rights? These questions need to be answered – at the beginning of the chapter – because of their impact on the development of the law. The chapter concludes with an outline of the child-care system, i.e. what happens when the normal workings of a family have broken down and social workers need to take action to protect a child from abuse or neglect.

Childhood and children's rights

There is a vast literature on the concept of **childhood** and continuing debate as to when children were first recognised and

Keywords

Childhood
A stage of human existence that is separate (and different) from that of adults; the state or period of being a child

treated as different from adults. In medieval times, for example, children worked and socialised alongside adults. Childhood was therefore much less distinct and special than it is now. But in the 17th century, attitudes towards children started to change. No longer regarded as their parents' property – who could be done with, more or less, as their parents wished – childhood began to be seen as a happy, carefree time.

However, it was the introduction of compulsory schooling in the late 19th century (which removed children from the workforce) and the scientific scrutiny of childhood (by the Child Study movement, formed in 1890) that most transformed attitudes towards children (Hendrick 1997a). These developments popularised the idea that children were different from adults in development, behaviour, knowledge, skills and in their dependence on adults (most often their parents). The 'discovery' of child cruelty and neglect at this time also prompted new concerns for the welfare of children.

In the 20th century other changes in society have similarly influenced our understanding of childhood. Smaller families, for example, have allowed deeper relationships between parents and their children (Moules 1998, p. 53). That children should have far greater opportunities for developing their decision-making capacities is also now widely accepted. As Fortin says (2003, p. 11): *'contemporary parents must accept that an important parental task is to provide children with conditions they need to develop into fully autonomous adults'*.

But this change in attitude, i.e. the idea that parents and other adults should promote children's capacity to make decisions for themselves, could not have happened without the influence of the children rights movement.

Children's rights

The notion of children's rights is a relatively modern one. It dates back to the Declaration of Geneva in 1924, which stated that 'mankind owes to the Child the best it has to give'. Several subsequent international documents also referred to children's rights in various situations but it was not until the 1989 UN Convention on the Rights of the Child that children were recognised as persons who were entitled to the same human rights as adults. As the first legally binding international document specifically about children, the Convention on the Rights of the Child has been enormously influential – indeed the touchstone for children's rights throughout the world (Fortin 2003, p. 49). It covers a wide range of rights – civil, political, economic and social – and has several aims, usually referred to as the 'four Ps' – prevention, protection, provision and participation.

But notwithstanding the influence of the Convention on the Rights of the Child the phrase 'children's rights' is problematic not least because it has been used in so many different ways. This means that translating children's human rights into legal rights has proved very difficult in practice. Writers who seek to do so usually take one or other of the following approaches:

Liberationist approach

Also known as 'kiddy libbers', liberationists (at least the most radical) want children to have same legal rights as adults. They therefore insist that children (of any age) should have, among other things, the right to vote, work for money, own and sell property, direct their own education, use drugs and so on. Not surprisingly, this extreme version of the liberationist approach has been criticised as unrealistic, impractical, reckless and potentially damaging to the family unit. However, even moderate liberationists, who demand far fewer rights and argue that children should only be banned from doing something because they are incompetent (rather than because of their age), are criticised – for ignoring the differences (physical and mental) between adults and children.

In summary, liberationists emphasise children's moral right to decide how to live their lives, i.e. to pursue their own vision of the 'good life'. Yet few writers who support this approach now claim complete personal autonomy for all children. What they are really claiming is for children to be given greater rights to self-determination than are currently allowed under the law. Or to put it another way, it is respect for the child's eventual capacity for autonomy, rather than autonomy now, that is important.

Welfare approach

The welfare view (also called 'protectionist') of children's rights focuses on making sure that children have access to adequate nutrition, housing, health care, education, a clean environment, financial support and so on. In seeking to protect children from inadequate care, neglect and abuse it also hopes to protect them from adult exploitation and oppression (such as pornography). Not surprisingly, 'welfarists' want the state to have a wide discretion to interfere in family life if a child is at risk. This is because they generally assume that children are vulnerable, ignorant, easily influenced and unable to make rational decisions. Paternalistic intervention in their lives is therefore justified. As a consequence, the welfare approach rarely leads to greater legal independence for children, nor much opportunity for them to exercise choice in health-care matters.

Reflective activity

Compare and contrast the liberationist and welfare view of children's rights.

Key points | Top tips

- Childhood is not a natural feature of human groups but is formed by social, historical, cultural and other factors
- The concept of children's rights can be used in different ways; two common approaches are the liberationist and welfare approach

Consent

The traditional legal approach in relation to consent and children was simple and convenient – parents were almost always seen as the appropriate people to decide what should happen to their children's bodies. But now that it is no longer acceptable to ignore children's capacity for choice or their right to be consulted and treated with respect, the law has had to change. Yet, as we shall see, despite the law's recognition that 'mature' children have a right to autonomy, the courts will overrule their wishes in certain circumstances. Similarly, in relation to young children the courts will generally authorise treatment parents have refused on the basis that children's lives are too precious to be sacrificed to their parents' beliefs.

Not surprisingly, the law distinguishes between children and young people who have capacity and those who are incompetent.

16- and 17-year-olds

Giving consent

Children in this age group have the same right to consent to treatment as adults, providing they are competent (i.e. able to comprehend and retain information and weigh it up – Family Law Reform Act 1969).

You should note the following:

- The word 'treatment' is widely defined in the Family Law Reform Act 1969 and so includes not just surgical, medical and dental treatment but also all nursing and other care
- Young people over 16 are (like adults) presumed to be competent (unless there is evidence to the contrary)
- An adolescent's valid consent cannot be overruled by anyone with parental responsibility (see the box below for who has parental responsibility)
- Only a court can overrule an adolescent's valid consent.

If the Act does not apply – because the 16- or 17-year-old is incompetent – consent can be given by a proxy. The proxy is almost always someone with parental responsibility (see box).

Who has parental responsibility?

The combined effect of the Children Act 1989 and the Adoption and Children Act 2002 is that the following have parental responsibility:

- Both parents, if they are married
- The mother, even if she is not married to the father
- The father who has made a parental responsibility agreement has been granted a parental responsibility order or has registered the birth jointly with the mother
- A step-parent (by agreement or court order)
- Adoptive parents
- 'Special' and ordinary guardians
- Other people who have parental responsibility because of a court order, e.g. a residence order granted to grandparents or a care order granted to the local authority.

Refusing consent

Competent 16- and 17-year-olds were once thought to have the same rights to refuse treatment as adults. But this appears not to be true. In a series of cases (e.g. *Re W* [1993], *Re M* [1999]) the courts have held that, even though such a refusal is a very important factor for health professionals to consider, it can be overruled by:

- Anyone with parental responsibility; or
- The court.

This means that competent children cannot effectively refuse treatment. It also means that reasonable force may be used to carry out treatment.

The difficulty with these cases is that they deny children under 18 the right to make a decision simply by reason of their age. Not surprisingly, liberationists are unhappy with this development. In contrast, those who adopt a more protectionist stance – and so are keen to protect young people from making self-destructive choices – welcome them. However, even those who adopt this paternalistic approach concede that forcing adolescents to have treatment that they have rejected may contravene the Human Rights Act 1998 (Fortin 2003, pp. 127–131).

Under-16-year-olds – 'Gillick-competent'

Giving consent

The law on giving consent for children under 16 was established in the famous Gillick case (*Gillick* v. *West Norfolk and Wisbech AHA* [1986]). A child who is '**Gillick-competent**' has an independent legal right to give consent to treatment. In assessing Gillick-competence you should consider the following questions:

- Does the child understand the nature of his/her medical condition, the proposed treatment, side effects and consequences of agreeing to or refusing treatment (see *Re L* [1998])?
- Does the child understand the moral, social and family issues involved? In *Re E* (1993), for example, the court did not think the 15-year-old understood the grief his parents would suffer if he died. He was therefore not Gillick-competent.
- How much experience of life does the child have? This question is particularly important if a child has been brought up by parents with strong religious views (such as Jehovah's Witnesses).
- Does the child's mental state fluctuate? If the child is competent at some times but not at others, the courts will consider him/her incompetent (*Re R* [1992]).
- How complex is the proposed treatment? The degree of understanding, intelligence and emotional and intellectual maturity required will inevitably vary depending on the complexity of the treatment and the associated risks. In other words, serious treatment requires a higher degree of maturity than routine treatments with few side effects.

Refusing consent

As to the right of Gillick-competent under-16-year-olds to refuse consent, there is no doubt that their informed refusal can be overruled by:

- Anyone with parental responsibility; or
- The court.

⊶ᴙ Keywords

Gillick-competent
Describes a mature minor under 16 who is competent to give consent without his/her parent's knowledge or permission

Over to you

Read Fortin 2003, pp. 72–74. Are you surprised by the research Fortin cites about children's capacity? If so, why?

Under-16-year-olds – not Gillick-competent

Children under 16 who are not Gillick-competent cannot give valid legal consent. Permission for treatment therefore has to come from someone else. This person (called a proxy) will usually be a parent (or other person with parental responsibility, see box on page 209).

For proxy consent to be lawful, treatment must be in the child's best interests. In most cases this is not problematic – despite the uncertainty of the phrase 'best interests' in relation to children (see box on page 212). But in disputes – such as when parents reject treatment that you or other health professionals strongly recommend – the courts are likely to be involved, especially when the child's life is at stake. In this kind of case the courts will usually follow medical opinion and so approve the recommended treatment – see, for example, *Re S* (1993) but contrast *Re T* (1997).

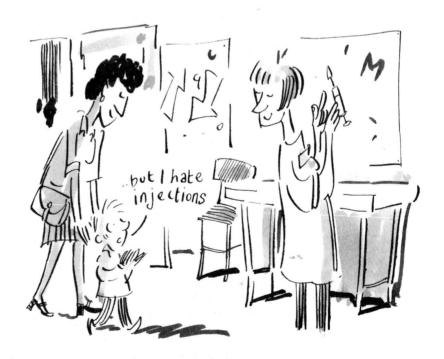

Consent for the young child is given by an adult with parental responsibility.

Top tips

- Be aware that in urgent cases any person currently caring for a child (such as a child minder) can give consent to treatment even though they do not have parental responsibility – Children Act 1989, section 3(5)

Definition of 'best interests' in relation to children

'Best interests' includes:

- Medical interests:
  - Nature of treatment
  - Chances of success
  - Its advantages and disadvantages
  - Suffering and risks
  - Quality of life.
- General interests:
  - Psychological needs
  - Family relationships
  - Educational benefits
  - Financial benefits.

See further the 'welfare checklist' in section 1(3) of the Children Act 1989.

Other aspects of the law relating to the care and treatment of children you should know are:

- Parents are not legally required to allow health professionals to monitor their children's health and development
- There is no legislation forcing parents to have their children vaccinated
- Parents can be guilty of criminal neglect if they wilfully fail to provide their child with adequate medical aid
- If parents fail to seek medical attention a social worker may intervene and take the child into care (see below)
- The courts are very unlikely to force you (or other health professionals) to provide treatment that you consider – having followed accepted practice – is inappropriate (*Re J* [1990]).

Top tips

- The Department of Health website: www.doh.gov.uk/consent/guidechild.htm contains useful guidance on children and consent

Key points *Top tips*

Unless there is a court order forbidding treatment you can treat a child if:

- The child is competent and consents to treatment; or
- Those with parental responsibility consent to treatment; or
- The court declares the treatment lawful; or
- The defence of necessity applies

Research

Mason *et al.* convincingly put the case for research on children:

> A child is by no means a miniature version of an adult. Children respond differently to drugs, as they do to a number of other treatments, and it is impossible to say that the effect of a particular therapy on an adult will be mirrored when applied to a child. Medical research on children is, therefore, necessary.
>
> Mason *et al.* 2002, p. 594

Although few people doubt the necessity of research involving children, such research can be problematic because there is always a danger that children will be used to further adult interests. The particular vulnerability of children explains why there are several influential ethical guidelines specifically relating to children. Currently the most detailed of these are those issued by the Royal College of Paediatrics and Child Health (2000).

Ethical guidance

In summary, the Royal College of Paediatrics and Child Health guidelines are based on the following principles:

- Research involving children is important for the benefit of all children and should be supported, encouraged and conducted in an ethical manner
- Children are not small adults, they have an additional, unique set of interests
- Research should only be carried out on children if comparable research on adults could not answer the same question
- All proposals involving medical research should be submitted to a research ethics committee
- Research that is not intended directly to benefit the child (i.e. is non-therapeutic) is not necessarily unethical or illegal.

In the absence of specific legislation governing research, the most important legal issue is consent (but see also NHS Research Governance, Chapter 8). The general principles of consent were explained in Chapter 6 (as were the consequences of acting without consent). In principal these apply equally to research, although there are special considerations, which we consider below.

Under-18-year-olds – Gillick-competent

Because of doubts as to whether the Family Law Reform Act 1969 covers research, most legal texts advise that only if children under 18 pass the Gillick test can they independently consent to research. Applied to research this means that they must be able to understand:

- The nature and purpose of the research, any possible risks and how great or small those risks are
- What will happen to them if they agree to enter the trial
- Whether the trial will directly benefit them (i.e. whether the research is therapeutic or non-therapeutic).

Other important things to note are:

- A relatively high standard of understanding and maturity would normally have to be reached (especially if the research is non-therapeutic)
- If a competent young person under 18 refuses to participate in research it is wise not to rely solely on parental consent, i.e. you should respect the mature minor's refusal (or alternatively seek the court's approval)
- Many legal texts advise against carrying out research with mature minors unless their parents also consent.

Under-18-year-olds – not Gillick-competent

As to children who are not Gillick-competent, consent must be obtained from a proxy – usually a parent or anyone else with parental responsibility, or a court. A proxy's powers in relation to research are wide, but do have limits. Thus if the research is therapeutic the proxy's consent will be lawful if it is in the child's best interests. As shown in the box on page 212, this term is broad enough to include a wide range of interests – bearing in mind that benefits of research must always outweigh the risks.

That said, if a child has a serious illness it may be reasonable for the proxy to consent to research even if the risks are significant – assuming, of course, that the child could benefit (either in the long or short term; Montgomery 2003, p. 364).

As regards non-therapeutic research, a proxy's consent is lawful only if risks to the child are minimal (i.e. no greater than the risks parents commonly expose their children to in everyday life). Examples of minimal risks are observational studies and single urine samples (other than by aspiration).

It is also worth noting that, even when children are not mature enough to make their own decisions about participating in research, most professional guidelines recommend obtaining their assent or agreement (in addition to the proxy's consent) to being involved. Assent simply means getting the child's permission.

Key points | Top tips

- Children who are Gillick-competent can give valid legal consent to research
- If children are not Gillick-competent consent to research must be obtained from a proxy (usually a parent)

Child protection

This final section outlines child protection law. It begins by briefly describing the basic principles of the Children Act 1989 – which is usually described as the most comprehensive reform of child law in living memory. The Act's welfare provisions are then discussed and the section ends with a summary of the main court orders that are available to protect children from neglect and abuse.

General principles of the Children Act 1989

The Children Act 1989 revolutionised childcare law. It replaced a confusing, complex and sometimes inconsistent system with a much more comprehensive code. At the same time it introduced sweeping changes to the law governing the circumstances in which local authorities could intervene compulsorily in the upbringing of a child. Designed to strike a 'new' balance between the role of the state, the rights of children and the responsibilities of parents, the Act was built on several fundamental principles. These include the following.

- **The welfare principle**. This is a 'golden thread' running through the Act. It emphasises that children come first and that their interests must be the paramount consideration whenever a court makes a decision about their upbringing.

- **Prevention rather than intervention – the primacy of the family**. The belief that children are best cared for by their families is reflected in many of the Act's provisions, which aim overall to ensure that the state only interferes in family life when it is absolutely necessary and the only way to protect children. Local authorities are therefore expected to do all they can to keep families together and children living at home. The themes of partnership, co-operation and support for families thus replace the emphasis on coercion that pervaded previous legislation.
- **The child's voice**. Throughout the Act there are sections that aim to improve children's legal status and capacity for independent action. Thus they are given greater rights – to be consulted, have their views taken into account and represented – than was previously the case.

Welfare services – supporting the family

Part III of the Act gives local authorities wide powers and duties to support families and help prevent parents 'losing' their children into state care. The overall aim of Part III is thus to keep families together. Almost all the services are targeted on a group of children considered especially vulnerable. These are so called 'children in need'. A child in need is one:

- Who is disabled
- Who is unlikely to achieve or maintain a reasonable standard of health or development without the provision of services
- Whose health or development is likely to be significantly impaired unless services are provided (see further section 17).

The services covered include accommodation, day care, advice, counselling, family centres and so on. Although well intentioned, there is ample evidence that Part III provision has been undermined by a shortage of resources. In other words, there are not enough social workers, homemakers, family aids, substitute carers or treatment resources (Fortin 2003).

Your role under Part 111

You are most likely to be involved in:

- Identifying and assessing which children are 'in need'
- Giving advice and guidance to prevent neglect and abuse (e.g. by teaching parenting skills and helping new parents understand the development needs of young children)
- Advising other agencies involved in child protection how a child's health needs can best be met.

Compulsory intervention – court orders

If providing support to a family fails to protect a child at risk, compulsory intervention may be necessary. Social workers can use a range of court orders. Some of these are temporary measures but others are long term (and give local authorities much more control over a child's life).

Before the court can grant any compulsory order, however, it has to be proved that a child 'is suffering (or likely to suffer) **significant harm**'.

The Act defines 'significant harm' (often referred to as the 'threshold criteria') in a complicated way. The intention is to make sure that the term is wide enough to cover every type of harm – i.e. damage to a child's physical or mental health and also the impairment of his or her physical, intellectual, emotional, social and behavioural development.

In practice what harm is 'significant' is not always clear – except when a child has been severely injured or neglected. Guidance emphasises that:

> There are no absolute criteria on which to rely when judging what constitutes significant harm. Consideration of the severity of ill-treatment may include the degree and the extent of physical harm, the duration and frequency of abuse and neglect, and the extent of premeditation, degree of threat and coercion, sadism, and bizarre or unusual elements in child sexual abuse.
>
> Department of Health 1999, para. 2.17

Short-term orders

These consist of the following:

Child Assessment Order

The Child Assessment Order (CAO; section 43) provides an opportunity to assess a child whose health or development is causing real concern but who is not thought to be in any immediate danger. The CAO lasts for 7 days (during which time the child may be removed from home).

Emergency Protection Order

The Emergency Protection Order (EPO; section 44) is designed for genuine emergencies when immediate protection is necessary. The EPO is one of the Act's most draconian compulsory powers. Among other things it not only allows the child to be removed from home but gives limited parental responsibility to local authorities – enough

○━┰ *Keywords*

Significant harm
Ill-treatment or the impairment of health or development which is considerable or important (section 31 of the Children Act 1989)

for social workers to consent to urgent medical examinations and/or treatment. An EPO can last for up to 15 days.

Police powers

The police may not only be involved in enforcing an EPO but can also initiate their own protective action. Section 46 gives them the right to remove children from home (and also to stop them from leaving hospital or other safe place). Although the police do not need the court's permission to use these powers (unlike the EPO and CAO), they are very short term – no longer than 72 hours.

Long-term orders

Long-term orders typically follow the above temporary measures. They should be used only if all other options (such as the provision of services) are inappropriate.

Care orders

Care orders give local authorities parental responsibility (which they share with parents). The effect of a care order is that social workers have considerable control over a child's upbringing. This means they can decide, for example, where the child should live, go to school, etc. Under a care order a child will normally (but not always) live away from home (either with foster carers or in a residential home). Children 'in care' may, however, return home on a trial basis – if the 'care plan' is for them to be rehabilitated with their families. Care orders can last until a child is 18 but they can be discharged before then.

Supervision orders

Supervision orders are ideal for less serious cases of neglect or abuse. They are also useful when a child is 'beyond parental control'. Supervision orders are shorter than care orders (lasting initially for 1 year). They do not give local authorities parental responsibility. Nevertheless, they do give them the power to supervise certain aspects of a child's upbringing. When imposing a supervision order the courts can include a wide range of health-related conditions. Supervision orders are not popular with practitioners.

Reflective activity

Do you think children who are abused or neglected always benefit from being removed from their families? If not, why not?

Your role in compulsory intervention

You are likely to be involved in the following ways:

- You may have concerns about a child, and refer those concerns to social services or the police
- You may be approached by social services and asked to provide information about a child or family
- You may be required to attend a child protection conference
- You may be asked to carry out a specific type of assessment, or provide help or a specific service to a child or member of their family
- You may be required to contribute to reviewing a child's progress.

Key points **Top tips**

- Local authorities have a legal duty to investigate suspected cases of child abuse (section 47, Children Act 1989)
- If you are working with children and families you must:
  - Be familiar with and follow your organisation's procedures and protocols
  - Remember that an allegation of child abuse or neglect can lead to criminal investigations
  - (When referring a child) consider and include relevant information you have on a child's developmental needs and his/her parent's/carer's ability to respond to those needs
  - Record all concerns, discussions about the child, decisions made and the reasons for those decisions
- You can find out more about what to do if you are worried a child is being abused on line at: www.doh.gov.uk/safeguardingchildren/index.htm
- Radical reforms to improve interagency co-ordination between, for example, local social workers, health professionals, the police and schools are contained in the Children Bill 2004 (available on line at: http://www/parliament.uk/index.cfm)

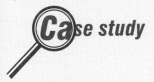 **Case study**

Karen's confidentiality

Karen is a mature 15-year-old who has been going out with her 18-year-old boyfriend for several months. She wants to go on the Pill but is reluctant to see her GP for fear that she will tell her mother.

Is Karen owed a duty of confidentiality?

Once an obligation to maintain confidentiality has arisen it is owed as much to children under 18 as it is to any other person, providing they are sufficiently mature to form a relationship of trust. What this means is that, irrespective of a child's competence to consent to treatment, the child is nonetheless owed a duty of confidence if they understand what it means to trust someone with secret

Case study continued

information. This is, however, subject to any relevant exception (see Chapter 7). Note too that even if requested treatment is refused the confidentiality of the consultation should still be respected (Hendrick, 1997b).

Put simply, competence and the duty of confidentiality are not necessarily connected even if in some cases, for example those involving very young children, they will be. In other words, they will be neither competent nor mature enough to understand what keeping a promise means. In such cases disclosure of information to parents may be an integral part of the child's care. Of course if children are Gillick competent then disclosure without their consent will not normally be lawful (see further Montgomery 2003, pp. 308–311).

Applying the above to Karen it is clear that she is owed a duty of confidentiality.

Rapid recap

Check your progress so far by working through each of the following questions.

1. What is the Gillick test?
2. Why is it important to know who has parental responsibility?
3. When can parents give consent to research on their children?
4. What does 'significant harm' mean?
5. When are children owed a duty of confidentiality?

If you have difficulty with more than one of the questions, read through the section again to refresh your understanding before moving on.

References

Department of Health (1999) *Working Together to Safeguard Children: A guide to inter-agency working to safeguard and promote the welfare of children*. HMSO, London.

Fortin, J. (2003) *Children's Rights and the Developing Law*. Butterworths, London.

Hendrick, H.J. (1997a) Constructions and reconstructions of British childhood: an interpretive survey, 1800 to the present. In: *Constructing and Reconstructing Childhood: Contemporary issues in the sociological study of childhood* (eds A. James and A. Prout). Falmer Press, London.

Hendrick, J. (1997b) *Legal Aspects of Child Health Care*. Chapman & Hall, London.

Mason, J.K., McCall Smith, R.A. and Laurie, G.T. (2002) *Law and Medical Ethics*, 6th edn. Butterworths, London.

Montgomery, J. (2003) *Health Care Law*. Oxford University Press, Oxford.

Moules, T. (1998) The growing child. In: Moules, T. and Ramsay, J. *Textbook of Children's Nursing*. Stanley Thornes, Cheltenham.

Royal College of Paediatrics and Child Health (2000) Guidelines for the ethical conduct of medical research involving children. *Archives of Disease in Childhood* **82** 177–182.

13

Caring for older people

Introduction

There are many ethical and legal issues associated with ageing but for the purposes of this chapter they can be conveniently grouped around three themes – autonomy, access to health and 'elder abuse'. These topics have been chosen because they bring sharply into focus the experience of growing old and so force us to consider how older people can retain their dignity, privacy and personhood even if their capacity to act, to remember or even to think clearly is severely diminished. We begin, however, with some facts about the ageing population and an exploration of society's attitude to older people.

Demographic changes – our ageing society

There is no doubt that Britain (like the much of the rest of the world) is getting older. Here are some statistics:

- The number of people over 65 has more than doubled since the early 1930s

- The number of people over 80 is set to increase by almost half (with the number of people over 90 doubling)

- For the first time ever there are more over-60-year-olds than under-16-year-olds

- By 2005 one person in five will be over 70 (Mason *et al.* 2002).

There are several explanations for this 'population time-bomb', such as the falling birth rate, contraception, the welfare state and a desire for smaller families. But arguably the most significant factor is rising **life expectancy**. That life expectancy has dramatically increased over the last century is beyond doubt – rising from around 45 years for males and 49 years for females in 1901 to over 75 and 80 respectively in 2000. Not surprisingly, increased life expectancy has significant implications for the NHS. Thus not only are older people the major users of health and social care (e.g. almost two-thirds of general and acute beds are used by people over 65) but also the pattern of this use has changed in recent decades. So, for many older people, particularly the most frail, the pattern of need is now of some level of continuing care, interspersed with acute episodes that require rapid access to medical treatment, nursing and therapy.

Other implications for the NHS arising from our ageing society can be gleaned from the following predictions and statistics:

- Notwithstanding wide differences in the social circumstances and economic status of older people, the number of people aged 65 or over who are suffering from long-standing illnesses (such as heart problems, arthritis, sight or hearing defects) will rise – from around 6 million today to over 9 million by 2036 (Mason *et al.* 2002, p. 389)
- That dementia also increases with age is similarly well known: affecting one in 20 of the population over 65 but one in five of those over 80 (McDonald and Taylor 1995, p. 5)
- The NHS currently spends 40% of its total budget on people over 65; this percentage will rise (as the percentage of over 65s in the population rises).

Key points **Top tips**

Remember that older people are not a uniform category but can be divided into the following distinct groups:

- **Entering old age**: includes those who have retired – either 'early' (i.e. from 50 onwards) or at the traditional age of 65
- **Transitional phase**: consists of those people who are in transition between healthy, active life and frailty
- **Frail old age**: vulnerable as a result of health problems such as stroke or dementia, social care needs or a combination of both.

Attitudes to older people

Ageism

The term **ageism** was coined in the 1960s to describe negative attitudes towards older people and the way they are portrayed as a social problem and a burden on society simply because they are 'old'. Ageism thrives because of common misconceptions that stereotype older people as 'out of touch with reality', confused, frail, senile, vulnerable, powerless and so on. The image of the older person in institutional settings is particularly negative – typically that of a person without a sense of self or identity and utterly dependent on others (Agich 1996, p. 146). These stereotypes are harmful, for two main reasons. First, they imply (wrongly) that older people can be treated as a group, regardless of their individual differences (physical and mental). Secondly, they reinforce the idea that older people are a relentless drain on limited resources, especially health care.

Discrimination

Discrimination exists in many areas of life and can prevent older people from accessing employment, goods and services (McDonald and Taylor 1995, p. 17). It also means that people's risk of receiving inadequate health care increases as they age – with, for instance, upper age limits for routine screening. Research in cardiology, for example, suggests that older people in particular are more likely to have more severe coronary heart disease, to be treated less vigorously and less effectively than younger people, to be treated medically rather than surgically and to be denied access to many cardiac facilities (Bowling *et al.* 2002, p. 188).

Tackling ageism in the NHS

The National Service Framework (NSF) for older people was published in 2001. It is an important document because it was the first time that the government had openly acknowledged the existence of age discrimination in the NHS. The National Service Framework emphasises the necessity of putting older people, their needs and those of their families and carers at the heart of policy and practice. Most importantly, it aims to stop age discrimination in health and social care by setting new national standards of care for all older people, whether they live at home or in residential care, or are being cared for in hospital.

The National Service Framework is a 10-year programme. In brief, the eight standards it sets are:

- **Rooting out age discrimination**. NHS services will be provided, regardless of age, on the basis of clinical need alone
- **Person-centred care**. NHS and social care services will treat older people as individuals – enabling them to make choices about their own care
- **Intermediate care**. Older people will have access to a new range of intermediate care services at home or in care settings to promote their independence

- **General hospital care**. Old people's care in hospital will be delivered through appropriate specialist care and by hospital staff who have the right skills to meet their needs
- **Strokes**. The NHS will take action to prevent strokes; people who are thought to have had a stroke will have access to diagnostic services and be treated by a specialist stroke service
- **Falls**. The NHS will take action to prevent falls and reduce resultant fractures or other injuries; older people who have fallen will receive effective treatment and rehabilitation
- **Mental health in older people**. Older people who have mental health problems will have access to integrated mental health services to ensure effective diagnosis, treatment and support for them and their carers
- **Promoting an active healthy life in older age**. The health and well-being of older people will be promoted through a co-ordinated programme of action.

Top tips

- You will find a comprehensive account of the nursing implications of the National Service Framework for older people in Nursing and Midwifery Advisory Committee's (2001) *Caring for Older People: A nursing priority*. The report is available on line at: www.doh.gov.uk/snmac/publications.htm

Key points

- To combat ageism in the NHS the National Service Framework for older people was set up in 2001
- The NSF sets eight new national standards of care; it means that decisions on treatment will be made on the basis of clinical need – not age

Autonomy

Ethical issues

For some people the potential loss of privacy and independence – both of which are the strongest expression of personal identity – they may experience as they grow older is their greatest fear. In Chapter 6 we discussed how our society places a very high value on autonomy and a person's ability to runs his/her own life. Indeed, it has been suggested that our fascination with independence explains why some people question the moral worth of those who no longer have the capacity to live independently or to make the kinds of decision they once took for granted (Campbell *et al.* 2001, p. 188). Expressed another way, the question is: Are individuals ravaged by the diseases and afflictions of old age, such as the loss of capacities associated with Alzheimer's disease, less worthy of our attention and care? Or do these individuals retain moral worth that transcends their frailties and demands special care and attention (Agich 1996, p. 142)?

Questions about the moral status of older people with diminished autonomy may require us to reconsider philosophical concepts such as the nature of personhood (Chapter 10). But in practice your main concern is likely to be how you can respect the respect the humanity and dignity of your patients but at the same time make decisions on their behalf (which may involve disregarding their choices or even not consulting them at all). There is, in short, the potential for conflict between autonomy on the one hand and paternalism on the other.

The dilemma posed by this conflict arises because if you are working with older people some of them may – to varying degrees – be unable to make or express choices or even understand what is happening to them. To get the balance right, i.e. to justify paternalistic intervention, the following points need to be stressed.

Few people are incapable of making any decisions at all

Even if patients have limited autonomy it does not necessarily mean that they are incapable of making any autonomous decision for themselves. So although one of your patients may not be able to understand the implications of complex surgery s/he may nevertheless still be able to make some choices about daily activities, such as personal hygiene, eating, clothing and so forth. Furthermore, even people with advanced dementia may be able to communicate in some way – through activities such as painting, photography, song and so on.

Fluctuating capacity

An individual's capacity to make decisions may vary depending on the environment, the people around them, the time of day, reaction to medication and so on. Promoting autonomy therefore means that, unless action is immediately necessary, you should delay decision-making until the 'right' moment, i.e. you should wait for a lucid (or sane) phase.

Assessing capacity

Older people are particularly vulnerable to having decisions about their care and treatment made for them simply because they are old.

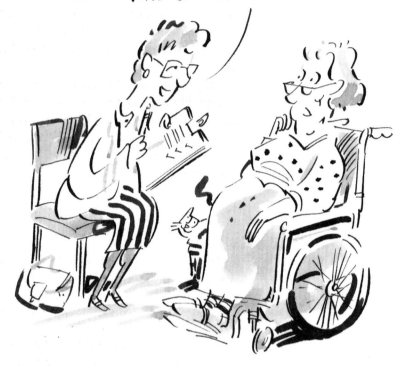

...and can you tell me who the Prime Minister is?

Assessing capacity.

In other words, assumptions are automatically made about their capacity without it actually being assessed. As a result they are more likely to become passive recipients of services rather than active participants in decisions about care. To resist the temptation to act paternalistically it is therefore vital that you assess capacity on a decision-specific basis, i.e. in the context of the activity that is to be decided. This means that, although a patient may be incapable of making a major decision – about whether to accept or refuse particular aspects of care, diagnosis or treatment – s/he may be able to make smaller decisions that lead to it (British Medical Association 1995).

Caring and treating older people who lack capacity

Once an elderly person has been assessed as incapable, paternalistic intervention – i.e. making choices on his/her behalf – can be justified, as long as these decisions are in their best interests. In some situations, e.g. giving a patient essential medication against his/her wishes or carrying out life-saving surgery, it may be relatively easy to justify acting in this manner. But what about more routine procedures such as basic care – e.g. when a patient refuses to wash or change his/her clothes? As Fletcher *et al.* note (1995, p. 167), forcing a patient to have a bath and change into clean clothes may be far harder to justify.

In practice whether such paternalistic intervention is ethically acceptable will depend on several factors, in particular whether the patient will harm himself (or others) if left unwashed and without clean clothes. Note too that sometimes it may be important to distinguish between nursing and personal care (although the boundaries between the two are not always clear).

Key points | **Top tips**

Ways in which you can promote the autonomy of older people include:
- Appreciating that incompetence in one area does not necessarily mean incompetence in another
- Working to understand their values and choices, in particular how they would wish to live their lives
- Never assuming that a older person's values are the same as yours
- Facilitating choices in as many aspects of daily life as possible, e.g. when to get up, what to eat, what to wear
- Providing information in an accessible manner – for example by writing it down so that poor memory can be overcome

---

Legal issues

The most important legal issue that arises in relation to caring for vulnerable older patients is consent. The position in law can be briefly summarised as follows:

Competent older patients

Competent older patients – those who can a) comprehend information relevant to a decision, b) retain this information and c) weigh it in the balance – have the same rights as other adults to consent to (and refuse) treatment and care (Chapter 6). Those with fluctuating capacity have similar rights, providing consent (or refusal) is sought when they are lucid. What this means is that the consent they gave during a sane period remains in force during subsequent incapacity, providing only a reasonably short time has elapsed between giving consent and the treatment being carried out. What is reasonable depends on the circumstances but it could be as long as 3 months (Dimond 2002, p. 385).

Incompetent older patients

No one currently has the power to give consent on behalf of an incompetent patient over 18. However, incompetent older patients (like other adult patients who lack capacity) can be treated without consent under the common law principle of best interests. Yet, as we saw in Chapter 11, the scope of the best interests test is unclear. Whether proposals in the Mental Capacity Bill 2004 will clarify the law remains to be seen. These will allow some decision-making powers to be given to various people (for day-to-day decisions, including health-care decisions). More serious health-care decisions could be referred to a court.

One of the most common situations you may face when caring for incapable elderly patients involves medication. As Dimond notes (2002, p. 389), there may be many occasions when, for a variety of reasons ranging from justifiable ones to pure cussedness or confusion, elderly patients may reject tablets, injections or liquids. What should you do? If the patient is competent his/her refusal must, of course, be respected. If not, then as long as the medication is essential and in the patient's best interests it can be given – but not before every possible effort has been made to persuade the patient to take it willingly (see further UKCC 2001).

Key points Top tips

- Competent older patients have the legal right to refuse treatment and care
- Incompetent older patients can be treated and cared for under the 'best interests' principle

Over to you

Read Mason *et al.* 2002, ch. 12 to find out:

- What legal options are available to remove incompetent elderly to a home or hospital
- The role of the Court of Protection.

Access to health care

It is widely accepted that it is not possible for the NHS to provide all the health care that is requested, i.e. supply exceeds demands. Health services therefore need to be rationed. How scarce health resources can be distributed fairly was explored in Chapter 3. The issue we consider here is whether age should be a factor in deciding who gets what. That this is an important question – with ethical and legal implications – is self-evident given our ageing society and the fact that, as people age, their use of the health service is likely to increase.

Consider the following simple example: two patients require a heart transplant and both are on the waiting list. In deciding who to treat first a hospital must choose between patient A – a 40-year-old head teacher of a large comprehensive school – and patient B – a 75-year-old who retired from his job as a school caretaker 15 years ago. Apart from their age and employment status there are no significant differences between them.

Who should be given the heart?

Ethical issues

Several approaches can be taken. Here we focus on those in which age may be a significant factor (see Chapter 3).

Quality-adjusted life years

The QALY approach places a value on the outcome of medical intervention according to the 'quality-adjusted life years' (QALYs) that would result. It aims to calculate the most efficient use of resources – that which will most improve the quality of people's lives over the longest period of time. Patients who score well on the QALY scale are those who are the cheapest to treat and who will achieve the best quality of life for the longest time.

This explains why, for example someone aged 75, who is likely to live for a further 5 or 7 years after treatment, is generally bound to lose out to a patient aged 40, who is expected to live for 20–30 years after the same treatment (Campbell *et al.* 2001, p. 181). In other words, older people are always likely to be at a disadvantage because their life expectancy is shorter than that of a younger person. Furthermore, as Herring points out (2001, p. 566), the QALY approach ignores the fact that some treatments may be necessary even though they score badly on the QALY scale (e.g. pain relief in the last few days of a person's life).

The fair innings argument

A related approach is the so-called 'fair innings' argument, i.e. that older people have had a fair (i.e. good) slice of the 'health-care cake' and so should give up their place in the queue to younger patients (who have not as yet had their chance to reach 'old age'). The major flaw in claiming that it is 'fair' for the old to make way for the young is that such an approach ignores the value each of us puts on our own lives. As Harris reminds us:

> All of us who wish to go on living have something that each of us values equally although for each of us it is different in character. . . . This thing is of course 'the rest of our lives'. So long as we do not know the date of our deaths then for each of us 'the rest of our lives' is of indefinite duration. Whether we are 17 or 70 . . . so long as we each wish to live out the rest of our lives . . . we each suffer the same injustice if our wishes are deliberately frustrated and we are cut off prematurely.
>
> Harris 1985, p. 89

Another objection to the 'fair innings' argument is that research strongly indicates that older people are in practice unwilling to give up their place to a younger person. In one important study, for example, people aged 65 and over were asked to imagine they had a heart condition that required surgery and that they were on an NHS waiting list. They were then asked if they would be prepared to give up their place on the cardiac surgery waiting list to a younger person (aged 45). The research revealed that the majority did not wish to cede priority on the waiting list to people younger than themselves (Bowling *et al.* 2002, 187–192).

The 'ageing is part of life' approach

Perhaps the most controversial of all approaches is the one developed by Daniel Callahan. In his ground-breaking book *Setting Limits* (1997) he argues that we can avoid older people increasingly being seen as a burden on society if we change our attitudes to old age and stop pretending that it can be turned into some form of endless middle age. We should, in short, accept ageing as an inevitable part of life rather than a medical obstacle to be overcome. So, instead of encouraging medicine to keep us alive at all costs – and possibly well beyond our 'natural lifespan' – we should be looking for ways of giving meaning to old age. As such we should value medicine that concentrates on the relief of pain and suffering for those at the end of their lives, thus improving their quality of life rather than striving heroically to extend it.

Predictably, Callahan's approach was widely condemned. Critics claimed that it was morally wrong to set limits on the elderly, who in any case cannot simply be dismissed as a group given the huge differences in their health status. Furthermore, the idea of a natural life span is too vague a concept to be at all helpful. And finally, the approach is unfair – because treatment decisions should be based only on individual need.

Reflective activity

Do you think age should be a factor in allocating scarce health resources? Should medical research concentrate less on life-prolonging technology and more on chronic problems of ageing such as incontinence and arthritis?

'Elder abuse'

Keywords

Elder abuse
In relation to older people this includes the ill-treatment or impairment of, or avoidable deterioration in, their physical or mental health, or the impairment of their physical, intellectual, emotional, social or behavioural development (Law Commission 1995)

Recognition that older people may be abused and neglected by their families as well as by outsiders dates from the mid-1980s. Although elder abuse is now much more widely recognised than it once was, the public is still probably not as aware as it should be – either of the extent of such abuse or its nature. In fact the degree of ignorance of – or, as some would say, indifference to – the problem has been compared to that which applied to child abuse 40 years ago (Mason *et al.* 2002, p. 390).

Defining elder abuse

Elder abuse is defined as *'the mistreatment of an older person ... it can be a single or repeated act or lack of appropriate action occurring within any relationship where there is an expectation of trust, which causes harm or distress to an older person'* (Action on Elder Abuse website 1995).

There are five main types of abuse (see box below).

Types of elder abuse
Examples of elder abuse are:
- **Physical**: hitting, slapping, burning, pushing, restraining or giving too much (or the wrong) medication
- **Psychological**: shouting, swearing, frightening, blaming, ignoring or humiliating a person

continued

- **Financial**: the illegal or unauthorised use of a person's property, money, pension book or other valuables
- **Sexual**: forcing a person to take part in any sexual activity without his/her consent – this can occur in any relationship
- **Neglect**: where a person is deprived of food, heat, clothing, comfort or essential medication.

Notes:

- An older person may suffer from only one form of abuse or from different types at the same time
- Abuse can occur by omission (i.e. failure to give proper care)
- Abuse can be unintentional – where someone is trying to help but acts in the wrong way through ignorance.

Source: Action on Elder Abuse website.

How much abuse occurs is difficult to gauge, largely because much abuse goes unreported. One influential study, however, suggested that up to 5% of older people in the community were suffering from verbal abuse and up to 2% were the victims of physical or financial abuse (Ogg and Bennett 1992). But a later study found a much higher level of abuse – that 27.5% of pensioners had been the victim of abuse or neglect (Ogg and Munn-Giddings 1993). Other important facts about elder abuse are that:

- Most abuse and neglect takes place at home (although about a quarter takes place in hospitals, nursing and residential homes)
- Three times as many women are abused as men
- Abuse appears to increase with age
- In a care setting abuse was most likely to be physical or neglect and to be perpetrated by a worker.

Anyone can be an abuser but the following are most likely to be in a position to mistreat an older person: a partner, child or relative; a friend or neighbour; a health-care, social-care or other worker; a volunteer worker.

Like other forms of abuse, elder abuse is a complex problem, not least because its causes are not yet fully understood. Nevertheless, although it can take many forms and range widely – from a spontaneous act of frustration to systematic premeditated assaults – certain risk factors have been identified. Those most associated with physical and psychological abuse are:

- Social isolation – those who are abused usually have fewer social contacts than those who are not abused

- There is a history of a poor-quality long-term relationship between the abused and the abuser
- A pattern of family violence exists – the person who abuses may have been abused as a child
- The person who abuses is dependent upon the person they abuse for accommodation, financial and emotional support
- The person who abuses has a history of mental health problems, a personality disorder or a drug or alcohol problem
- In care settings abuse may be a symptom of a poorly run establishment. It seems that it is most likely to occur where staff are inadequately trained, poorly supervised, have little support from management or work in isolation (Bennett and Kingston 1993, Decalmer and Glendenning 1997).

Ethical issues

Autonomy

One of the main ethical issues raised by abuse of older people is the principle of autonomy. As should now be clear, autonomy is a multilayered term. Broadly, it means respecting the choices people make concerning their own lives. When caring for older people, respecting autonomy may mean that the state is reluctant to remove adults from their homes or prevent them seeing someone simply because it is 'good for them'. In other words the following dilemma arises: how can you respect the autonomy of a victim of abuse (who may prefer to be cared for by an abusive relative) but at the same time adequately protect him/her (which may require moving him/her to a residential home)? Or, to put it another way, should the state act paternalistically and deprive an older person of his/her choice of how and where to live?

The obvious solution is to argue that it all depends on whether the victim is competent to make a decision. However, as we saw above, there may be real difficulties in assessing the competence of older people, especially if their understanding fluctuates from day to day. The other problem is of course whether we can be sure that the victim will always be better off living away from home.

A related problem is the difficulty of defining abuse and neglect. Thus, as we shall see in the case study on page 235, the boundaries between justifiable restraint and abuse are not always clear. And what about a carer who is irritable with an elderly patient? Some might regard ill-temper as an inevitable (and understandable) part of the stresses involved in providing personal care – especially if the carer is desperate, exhausted and solely responsible for the victim's well-being. Others might define it as abuse (Herring 2004).

Confidentiality

Another dilemma you may face is this: suppose you suspect that an elderly patient – living at home or in a residential or nursing home – is being abused, but she refuses to allow you to report the abuse? Should you report it anyway even though you have not been given consent to do so? In deciding what to do you will need to find out, as sensitively as possible, why the patient has refused to let you disclose the abuse. Perhaps she fears the abuse will get worse or refuses out of sense of loyalty, guilt or even responsibility. Either way, in reaching a decision you will need to follow all relevant guidance, i.e. your professional code of conduct, local standards, policies and procedures, and national guidelines on elder abuse.

The combined effect of this guidance requires you to:

- Always listen to what your patient is telling you
- Make sensitive enquiries in a safe, private environment
- Seek advice from a lead agency (e.g. social services, the police)
- Report any incident or suspicions to a lead agency
- Monitor the situation carefully
- Keep formal detailed accurate records of your information and observations
- Initiate emergency intervention if the patient requires removal to a place of safety by involving other agencies (such as arranging a doctor's visit about hospital or residential care).

Legal remedies

Although there is no legal duty on local authorities to investigate suspected elder abuse (as there is for children under the Children Act 1989), there is a range of remedies that aim to protect victims and prevent abuse. Both these strategies can involve either criminal or civil law.

Several types of criminal action can be brought against abusers under, for example, the Offences Against the Person Act 1861 and the Protection from Harassment Act 1997. But prosecutions are rare – either because the police are unaware of the abuse or because the victim is unable or reluctant to report it. Civil orders are also available (under the Family Law Act 1996). These include the non-molestation order – ordering the abuser not to 'molest' the victim' – and occupation order – which can remove the abuser from the victim's home. But the Act is complex and may be of very limited use if the abuse is occurring in a residential setting.

Note too the effect of the National Health Service and Community Care Act 1990, which requires local authorities to assess elderly people who may be 'in need of community services'. There is also a limited power under the National Assistance Act 1948 to remove a person from his/her home if s/he is living in insanitary conditions and not receiving proper care and attention. Legislation governing the registration and inspection of residential and nursing homes may similarly be relevant. For example, under the Care Standards Act 2000 local authorities have the right to enter and inspect homes and cancel or refuse registration.

Top tips

Useful websites on elder abuse are:

- Action on Elder Abuse: www.elderabuse.org.uk
- National Care Standards Commission: www.carestandards.org.uk
- Age Concern: www.ageconcern.org.uk

Key points

- Elder abuse can be physical, sexual, psychological, financial; it also includes neglect
- Autonomy and confidentiality are the main ethical and legal issues raised by elder abuse
- The law provides a number of routes to protect an older person from abuse

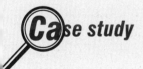

Case study

Wandering Derek

Derek is an 80-year-old widower. He suffers from dementia and, although physically strong and fit, he has become increasingly unable to carry out simple tasks such as dressing and feeding himself. His long-term memory is now very patchy – he does not believe he has ever been married or has children. In fact he was married for 30 years and has one son, Graham. He has lived with Graham for the last 2 years. Derek spends 3 days a week at a small Elderly Mentally Ill Assessment Unit.

Derek is very mobile and is known to wander. Constantly on the move, he rarely sits still for longer than 10 minutes at a time. Graham usually copes well with his restless behaviour and his wandering – by locking the front door, structuring his day and keeping him as busy as possible. But a few weeks ago Derek managed to unlock the front door and wandered into town. He just managed to cross a busy road but then got lost and became very distressed. Fortunately he was seen by a neighbour, who called Graham to pick him up.

Derek's wandering has now become a problem, particularly at the unit, where he is becoming very difficult to contain. Luckily Derek usually returns to the unit when approached but recently he has become aggressive when he is retrieved. Graham suggests that some form of restraint should be used.

Case study continued

**ꟻlɿeꟻ*Reflective activity*
1. Define 'wandering' and 'restraint'.
2. Consider the legal and ethical implications of using restraints.

1. Definitions

- **Wandering**. *'A tendency to move about either in a seemingly aimless or disoriented fashion, or in a pursuit of an indefinable or unobtainable goal'* (Stokes 1988) – it is one of the most important behavioural changes in dementia.

- **Restraint**. In broad terms, restraint means restricting someone's behaviour to prevent harm, either to the person being restrained or to other people – forms of restraint include harnesses, cot sides, locked rooms, tagging, boundary alarms and drugs.

2. Issues raised by restraints

Ethical issues

When considering the use of restraints the following principles should be kept in mind:

- The purpose of restraints should be to allow people the maximum amount of freedom and privacy compatible with their own safety

- The method used should always be the minimum possible in the circumstances and should be used only for as long as is necessary to end, or reduce significantly, the threat to the patient or to other people

- Where any form of restraint is proposed to protect mentally incapacitated people from harming themselves, it should be used only to the extent of preventing risk beyond that which would normally be taken by a similarly frail, mentally alert person

- Restraint should never be used simply to aid the smooth running of a unit or when there are too few staff on duty (British Medical Association 1995, see also Royal College of Nursing 1999).

Legal issues

Restricting a person's movement without lawful authority so that they have no way of escape is a form of false imprisonment and is therefore illegal (Dimond 2002, p. 387). Under common law, however, it is lawful to use temporary restraint providing that is the only way to prevent the patient injuring him/herself or someone else. But this common law power must be used sparingly – in other words, only in emergencies and when it is in the best interests of a mentally incapable patient (McDonald and Taylor 1995, p. 131). Furthermore, whatever restraint is used it must be both necessary and proportionate to the harm to be avoided.

Applying the above to Derek, several questions must be answered.

Case study continued

When considering the use of restraints the following principles should be kept in mind:

● Is Derek at risk, either immediately or in the longer term?
● Are others at risk from his behaviour?
● If the answer to either of the above is yes, can Derek be persuaded to change his behaviour?
● Have all other ways of managing his wandering (without using restraint) been considered and tried?

Depending on the answers to these questions, restraining Derek may be both ethically acceptable and lawful.

Reflective activity

Do you think the way wandering is defined in the case study is helpful? How would you define 'wandering'?
   Think about ways in which Derek's wandering could be managed.

Rapid recap

Check your progress so far by working through each of the following questions.

1. What does the word 'ageism' mean?
2. What is the National Service Framework for older people?
3. What is the 'fair innings' argument?
4. What is elder abuse?
5. Is it lawful to restrain a 'wandering' incompetent older person?

If you have difficulty with more than one of the questions, read through the section again to refresh your understanding before moving on.

References

Agich, G.J. (1996) Ethics and aging. In: *Birth to Death: Science and bioethics* (eds D.C. Thomasma and T. Kushner). Cambridge University Press, Cambridge.

Bennett, G. and Kingston, P. (1993) *Elder Abuse: Concepts, theories and interventions*. Chapman & Hall, London.

Bowling, A., Mariotto, A. and Evans, O. (2002) Are older people willing to give up their place in the queue for cardiac surgery to a younger person? *Age and Ageing* **31** 187–192.

British Medical Association (1995) *The Older Person: Consent and care*. BMA, London.

Callahan, D. (1997) *Setting Limits*. Georgetown University Press, Washington, DC.

Campbell, A., Gillett, G. and Jones, G. (2001) *Medical Ethics*, 3rd edn. Oxford University Press, Oxford.

Decalmer, P. and Glendenning, F. (eds) (1997) *The Mistreatment of Elderly People*. Sage, London.

Department of Health (2001) *National Service Framework for Older People*. HMSO, London.

Dimond, B. (2002) *Legal Aspects of Nursing*, 3rd edn. Pearson Education, Harlow.

Fletcher, N., Holt, J., Brazier, M. and Harris, J. (1995) *Ethics, Law and Nursing*. Manchester University Press, Manchester.

Harris, J. (1985) *The Value of Life: An introduction to medical ethics*. Routledge, London.

Herring, J. (2004) *Family Law*, 2nd edn. Pearson Education, Harlow.

Law Commission (1995) *Report 231: Mental incapacity*. HMSO, London.

McDonald, A. and Taylor, M.E. (1995) *The Law and Elderly People*. Sweet & Maxwell, London.

Mason, J.K., McCall Smith, R.A. and Laurie, G.T. (2002) *Law and Medical Ethics*, 6th edn. Butterworths, London.

Ogg, J. and Bennett, G. (1992) Elder abuse in Britain. *British Medical Journal* **305** 998–999.

Ogg, J. and Munn-Giddings, M. (1993) Researching elder abuse. *Ageing and Society* **13** 389.

Royal College of Nursing (1999) *Restraint Revisited: Rights, risk and responsibility, 000998*. Royal College of Nursing, London.

Stokes, G. (1988) Choosing the path to guide the wanderer. *Geriatric Medicine Community Nursing Supplement* 13–14.

UKCC (2001) *Covert Administration of Medicines*. United Kingdom Central Council for Nursing, Midwifery and Health Visiting, London.

Death, dying and the incurably ill patient

Learning outcomes

By the end of this chapter you should be able to:

- Understand the moral and legal principles that guide decision-making at the end of life
- Critically assess the arguments for and against euthanasia
- Describe the legal and ethical duties owed to the dying and incurably ill.

Introduction

Because of the enormous value we place upon life it is not surprising that the treatment of terminally or incurably ill patients is one of the most hotly debated issues in health care. The care of such patients has, of course, always raised acute dilemmas but decision-making at the end of life is now much more difficult than it once was. We begin this chapter by asking why this is so. We then explain some key terms used in the euthanasia debate before looking at the arguments for and against euthanasia. But the main focus of this chapter is a discussion of the ethical and legal principles that guide end-of-life decision-making. As you will see, this involves considering some of the most morally difficult issues you are likely to face, such as whether there is an obligation to prolong life at all costs, and whether there is a distinction between killing and letting die (and between foreseeing and intending death). This chapter also discusses the legality of DNAR ('do not attempt resuscitation') orders and advance directives. For reasons of space we cannot consider organ transplantation (on which see Montgomery 2003, ch. 19).

Why is caring for patients at the end of their lives more difficult now than it was in the past?

The care that patients receive at the end of their lives is now particularly contentious for several reasons. Here are some:

Attitudes to dying

According to Tschudin (2003, p. 141), nurses and doctors often have very different views as to the most appropriate care for patients who are terminally ill. Thus doctors may, for example, prescribe tests and treatments that they consider necessary but which nurses – who are more likely to know the patient's wishes – consider inappropriate. However, as Tschudin points out, even though different views about the care of patients who are dying or incurably ill may be inevitable at this time such professional rivalries can only harm patients.

Improved social conditions

Social conditions, at least in the Western world, have had a huge impact on the kinds of death people now typically experience. Thus in the early 20th century people died from, for example, kidney failure, heart attacks and infectious diseases. But where once these diseases were invariably fatal (and were commonly described as 'the old man's friend') they are now treatable (Cranford 1996, p. 191). Yet the control that modern technology has given us over death can be a two-edged sword. This is because the power of medicine to prolong lives and postpone death means that we face more profound dilemmas than we ever did in the past. Is it, for example, unquestionably beneficial to extend the life of a profoundly handicapped baby with no hope of recovery or improvement?

Changes in health care

Given the advances in modern medicine it is not surprising that the actual process of dying is very different now from the way it was in the past. Thus in the early part of the 20th century it was not uncommon for people to die at home surrounded by family, friends and a doctor who knew them well. But now, as Cranford points out (1996, p. 190), the typical deathbed scene is more likely to be in an institution surrounded by high technology and specialists (familiar with that technology but strangers to the person who is dying and his/her values). Is such a death, Cranford asks, the modern version of a 'good' death?

High profile cases

Practices once left mainly to doctors are increasingly being brought out in to the open by a series of high profile cases that make the headlines. Consider, for example, the case of Anthony Bland, the young man injured in the Hillsborough football stadium disaster who was in a persistent vegetative state for several years (see below). Another case during the same period (the early 1990s) was the trial of Dr Cox, who was charged with the attempted murder of one of his patients of 13 years' standing (whom he admitted he had injected with two ampoules of potassium chloride). But the most poignant recent case was that of Diane Pretty in 2001. Suffering from motor neurone disease and just able to communicate, she sought the court's assurance that her husband would not be charged with assisted suicide if he helped her to end her life. She failed to get the assurance she wanted but her plight generated a huge public debate about the rights of terminally ill people to choose the manner and time of their death.

Changing medical relationships

Changing medical relationships in a less paternalistic age, especially the expectation that patients should be consulted about their treatment, have increased the opportunities for disputes to arise. This explains why patients (and their carers) are more likely to challenge decisions by health cases on a wide range of end-of-life issues (e.g. resuscitation policies, life-saving treatment for profoundly disabled babies and so on).

Definitions

Many of the issues examined in this chapter involve, directly or indirectly, the following key terms: euthanasia, assisted suicide, death and medical treatment.

⚷ Keywords

Euthanasia
From the Greek *eu thanatos,* meaning good or easy death

Euthanasia

The word **euthanasia** originated in Greece and means a good or easy death. Nowadays the word is more often used to describe the deliberate ending of life. Several different types of euthanasia are usually recognised (see box below).

Types of euthanasia

- **Voluntary euthanasia**: a competent person makes an informed and free decision to end his/her life
- **Non-voluntary euthanasia**: a decision is taken to end a person's life because s/he is hopelessly or terminally ill; it is non-voluntary because the person cannot be consulted about the decision – s/he may be unconscious, for example, or too ill to make a choice
- **Involuntary euthanasia**: ending someone's life either without regard to their wishes, when they are competent to give them, or against their expressed wishes, supposedly in their best interests
- **Assisted suicide**: someone (typically a health professional) supplies the patient with the means – e.g. a lethal dose of drugs – to take his own life
- **Active euthanasia**: a positive action is taken to end life, e.g. administering a lethal injection
- **Passive euthanasia**: involves allowing a patient to die by omitting to act, e.g. by withholding (or withdrawing) life-saving treatment such as artificial nutrition or hydration.

Death

In the past death was a relatively straightforward state to identify and define. Thus when a person's heart or breathing stopped it was generally accepted that s/he was dead. While this definition remains adequate it is not appropriate when intensive treatment has been used to maintain a person's vital functions. To deal with such cases a different definition of death was developed, namely **brainstem death**. Although widely now accepted as the standard for determining death, the concept of brain death has always been controversial (Mason *et al.* 2002, ch. 13). Brainstem death has not been incorporated into legislation but it has been accepted by the courts (*Re A.* [1992]).

Medical treatment

Following the Bland case (see page 255) it is clear that life-sustaining treatment and medical support measures, such as artificial nutrition and hydration through the use of nasogastric tubes, percutaneous endoscopic gastrostomy, intravenous lines and so forth, are forms of medical treatment. As such they are no different from other forms of treatment (and so can be withheld or withdrawn in certain circumstances).

Keywords

Brainstem death
(Sometimes called whole-brain death or just brain death) the irreversible loss of brain function

---

Key points / Top tips

Be aware that:

- Feeding by 'normal means' is not normally regarded as medical treatment
- 'Normal means' refers to 'oral' nutrition and hydration, where food or drink is given by mouth

---

Arguments for and against euthanasia

This section considers some of the main arguments for and against euthanasia. As you will see, there are a wide range of viewpoints, ranging from a liberal approach (based on the autonomy principle) to the absolutist sanctity of life prohibition.

Arguments for euthanasia

Autonomy

The most persuasive argument in favour of euthanasia is the principle of autonomy. As we saw in Chapter 6, this principle requires you to respect your patients' rights to make their own decisions about their care and treatment. For some patients this right to self-determination might mean the right to choose death. The 'right to die' (as this 'right' is usually called nowadays) has become a more frequent demand in recent years. Most people (not surprisingly, considering how the phrase is represented in the media) assume that it refers to a decision – by terminally or incurably ill patients – that they do not want further treatment. Yet the phrase 'right to die' can be interpreted in another (less autonomous) way in this context – as a 'duty to die'. A 'duty to die' refers to terminally ill people who feel that they have no choice but to refuse treatment, because of social and other pressures – that they are, for example, a burden on their family or too costly to society (Tschudin 2003, p. 136).

Voluntary euthanasia is the easiest to justify on autonomy grounds – because it is based on a patient's free and informed choice. Non-voluntary euthanasia, on the other hand, is harder to justify – because then the decision to die is made by someone other than the patient him/herself (who is incompetent). Unless, that is, the so-called 'substituted judgement test' is used. This test (unlike the best interests one) is based on what the patient him/herself would have wanted, regardless of what others may think is a 'good' outcome. As an approach to decision-making it can be described as autonomous because it looks at the situation from the patient's point of view rather than the viewpoint of others (Kennedy and Grubb 2000).

The right to dignity

An argument closely related to autonomy is concerned with maintaining a person's dignity, in particular the right to die with dignity. The idea of 'death with dignity' has become a popular slogan in recent years, but what does it mean? Usually, the argument goes something like this: although medicine can now provide the means of staving off death, the cost to the individual may be too high. In other words, what patients think about life-sustaining technology is very important. Some may not, for example, want to spend their last days, weeks or months attached to tubes, drips and so on. What needs to be recognised, therefore, is that, even if in most cases the pain of those who are terminally ill can be controlled, what they may fear most is the technology that threatens their 'personhood', i.e. leads to a loss of self-respect, personal integrity and self-esteem.

Clearly, this type of argument implies that removing life support is the same as letting a person die with dignity. Yet, as Johnstone warns (1999, pp. 240–243), such a view assumes that the term 'dignity' has a clear-cut common-sense meaning. However, she asserts that this is not the case, since dignity is a subjective term (and so may mean different things to different people and different things to the same person at different times in his/her life). Note too that it is important to remember that, when people ask for death with dignity, they are not necessarily asking for euthanasia. Rather they may see this as the only dignified alternative to a death that has been 'taken over by medicine' (Cassell 1996, p. 222).

Reflective activity

What do the terms dignity and dying with dignity mean to you?

Actual practice

A more practical argument supporting euthanasia is that it is practised anyway. Thus, in one of many studies that have been carried out over the last few years – both on attitudes to and the practice of euthanasia – it was revealed that 22 out of 750 doctors admitted to having actively ended the life of a patient on request and a surprising 46% said they believed they should be legally permitted to do so (Mason *et al.* 2002, p. 548). Nevertheless very few doctors who have taken part in some form of euthanasia are prosecuted for murder, and those who are are almost always treated sympathetically by the courts and so are usually found not guilty. Given that euthanasia is practised behind closed doors, would it not be better, so the argument goes, to regulate it properly, thus ensuring that health professionals and patients are protected?

Arguments against euthanasia

Sanctity of life doctrine

One of the most popular arguments against euthanasia is the sanctity of life doctrine. There are different versions of this doctrine (which will be examined in more detail below), but it can be summed up as follows: human life is sacred and taking it is wrong; euthanasia is an example of taking human life; therefore euthanasia is wrong. Those who adopt this version of the doctrine insist that, whenever possible, human life should be maintained. This means that generally they are keen to put enormous resources into prolonging a person's life irrespective of the burden to that person or society.

Slippery slope argument

Another very persuasive objection to euthanasia is the so-called 'slippery slope' argument. It is an argument that has many forms (often it is called the 'thin end of the wedge' or 'tip of the iceberg'). But the main thrust of the approach is the claim that once we begin to kill others who have requested death, we will find ourselves sliding down a slope that leads to killings that no one wants (Singer 1995, p. 150). Or, to put it another way, our moral standards will inevitably drop as we move from voluntary euthanasia to compulsory euthanasia. So, although to begin with strict controls would be put in place to ensure, for example, that only those in uncontrollable pain would have their request for euthanasia carried out, gradually those controls would be relaxed. Euthanasia would then be extended not just to those who are incapable of requesting it but also to those who are not terminally or even chronically ill but have simply become too much of a burden for their families or society. And finally, it will not be long before people would simply be killed because their lives are considered unworthy.

Risk of abuse

Related to the slippery slope argument is the claim that, even if it were possible to draw appropriate boundaries and legalise euthanasia, it would never be possible to provide sufficient safeguards to prevent abuse. There is the very real risk, in short, that vulnerable people would be forced by unscrupulous relatives into making premature decisions they did not really want.

Discrimination

It is sometimes suggested that euthanasia is discriminatory because it implies that some lives are of less value than others and so are not worth prolonging. In other words, euthanasia discriminates against those who are terminally or incurably ill by reinforcing the idea that their lives, unlike others, are unimportant. According to this approach, then, just as any other act of discrimination is morally wrong, so too is euthanasia.

Key points *Top tips*

- Arguments in support of euthanasia include a) the autonomy principle, b) right to 'dignity' and c) actual practice
- Arguments against euthanasia include a) the sanctity of life doctrine, b) the slippery slope argument, c) risk of abuse and d) discrimination

Over to you

Read Johnstone 1999, ch. 12.
Overall do you think the arguments for or against euthanasia are the most persuasive? List your reasons.

Professional guidelines – good practice in decision-making at the end of life

There have been several attempts in recent years to introduce legislation on euthanasia but none has been successful. It is therefore not surprising that various professional bodies have issued comprehensive guidance on the basic moral principles that should guide practice. These cover withholding and withdrawing treatment as well as cardiopulmonary resuscitation. The most important current guidelines are Royal College of Paediatrics and Child Health (1997), General Medical Council (2002) and British Medical Association (2001a, b).

Although these guidelines vary in emphasis, several key moral principles emerge. In summary these are:

- Treatment of patients should reflect the dignity of every person, irrespective of age, debility, dependence, race, colour or creed
- Actions must reflect the needs of the patient as well as their values, beliefs and priorities
- Life has a natural end
- Prolonging a patient's life usually, but not always, provides a health benefit to that patient but it is not an appropriate goal of medicine to prolong life at all costs with no regard to its quality or the burdens of treatment
- Although emotionally it may be easier to withhold treatment than to withdraw it, there is no morally relevant difference between the two actions.

Making end-of-life decisions

This section begins by considering what many claim is both the starting point and most fundamental question in this context: is there an ethical and legal obligation to prolong life? We then describe the legal and ethical duties owed to patients who are terminally and incurably ill. Some very important distinctions are then explored, between killing and letting die, and between foreseeing and intending death.

Is there an obligation to prolong life?

In examining whether there is an ethical and legal obligation to prolong life we need to consider two approaches that are commonly used in the euthanasia debate – the sanctity of life doctrine and the quality of life approach.

Ethical aspects

Sanctity of life

The **sanctity of life** doctrine has a long history in Western thought. Traditionally, its roots lie in the Judaeo-Christian belief that human life is valuable and worthy of respect irrespective of its quality. As a gift from God, life is 'on loan' and thus not ours to do what we like with. Only God, therefore, has the right to take life away. From this it follows that any intentional act to end life, which interferes with the will of God, is morally wrong.

The belief that life is sacred in a religious sense may of course be less acceptable in our more secular society. Yet there is still widespread support for the principle that it is wrong to kill even though contemporary attitudes towards the sanctity of life doctrine (or 'right to life', which is how the doctrine is often described) are more varied (and complex) than in the past. Thus nowadays many people who believe instinctively that it is wrong to take human life do nevertheless concede that in some circumstances it can be justified. On the other hand, others still hold the extreme view of the doctrine – that human life must be preserved whatever the cost and whatever the circumstances.

According to some philosophers, however, even in its strongest form the sanctity of life doctrine does not claim that life is an absolute good and therefore one to which all others must be sacrificed. Keown (1997), for example, argues that the doctrine should be understood as meaning that life may never be intentionally taken. It is that principle that is absolute rather than the idea that life must be prolonged at all costs. Or, to put it another way, life-prolonging treatment is not always the overriding priority, as there may be some circumstances when death can be permitted. The difficulty lies, of course, in determining what those circumstances are, since it involves asking a question that is almost

⚷🖈 Keywords

Sanctity of life
The belief that human life is valuable for its own sake and that it is therefore morally wrong to deliberately end it

impossible to answer: when is life worth living? Or, to put it another way: what qualities of life make a life worthwhile?

Keywords

Quality of life
The belief that human life is valuable for its own sake and that it is therefore morally wrong to deliberately end it

Quality of life

Although the notion of **quality of life** is a popular one that many see as the central consideration when making life and death decisions, there is no widely accepted definition of the term. Indeed, as any examination of the literature quickly reveals, there are as many different interpretations of the concept as there are authors. But despite the difficulty of pin-pointing the essence of the concept Johnstone (1999, p. 366) suggests when thinking about quality of life most people use the term in one of the following three ways:

- **Descriptively**. This involves identifying certain traits or features a person might have, such as the patient is 'in pain' or 'is totally dependent on others'.
- **Evaluatively**. Here some value is attached to a particular trait or characteristic, i.e. the pain suffered by the patient is 'bad' or regaining independence is 'good'.
- **Prescriptively**. A prescriptive statement involves a moral judgement – a typical example would be: 'a life of such pain is not worth living' or 'being so dependent it is not in the patient's best interests to go on living'.

In the light of these different senses of quality of life it is self-evident that the potential for making 'moral errors' when deciding quality-of-life matters in health-care settings is enormous. It is also important to remember that people can have very different attitudes to the various characteristics that are usually regarded as constituting a 'quality of life', i.e. degree of pain and suffering, what it means to be healthy, ill, happy, to function effectively (socially, emotionally and physically), to be valued and respected, and so forth. Self-evident too is the fact that things that were important once in a person's life may change over time, becoming more or less significant as they age.

Despite the difficulty of defining the term quality of life precisely, if we accept it as a relevant consideration then it can at least be argued that there is no absolute ethical obligation to prolong life at all costs.

Legal aspects

The principle of the sanctity of life is a fundamental legal principle that is now enshrined in the Human Rights Act 1998 (Article 2). The courts have also repeatedly confirmed it – most recently in *Re S* (1995), *Re D* (1997) and *Re G* (2001). But the principle is not an absolute legal one. Thus, even though the law clearly prohibits taking active steps to terminate life, it does not require every patient to be resuscitated (or maintained on life support indefinitely – see, for example, *Re J* [1990], *Re C* [1998] below). Note too that the courts have also recognised that Article 3 of the Human Rights Act 1998 (the prohibition on torture, and cruel and inhuman treatment) encompasses the right to die with dignity (*D* v. *United Kingdom* [1997]).

In effect, then, the law recognises what has been called a 'qualified' sanctity of life principle (Stauch *et al.* 2002). It is qualified because according to the law a person's quality of life might be such that it is not in his/her best interests to prolong it. As the House of Lords said in the Bland case: 'the doctor who is caring for a patient cannot be under an absolute obligation to prolong life by any means available to him, regardless of the quality of the patient's life. Common humanity requires otherwise, as do medical ethics and good medical practice'.

Key points Top tips

- There is no legal or ethical obligation to prolong life whatever the cost and whatever the circumstances

Key points **Top tips**

When considering the sanctity of life doctrine and quality of life approach you must:

- Find out which life-sustaining technology a person does or does not want
- Find out the personal values of that person
- Be aware of how cultural, societal, spiritual and family values influence attitudes and beliefs to death and dying
- Be aware that risks and benefits of life-sustaining treatment vary with age, health condition and other factors such as pain

What duties are owed to the terminally and incurably ill?

In this section we consider the ethical and legal duties owed to the terminally and incurably ill. Ethical guidance is mainly derived from professional guidelines (see above). The law has mainly evolved from case law (rather than legislation).

To act in patients' 'best interests'

Ethical aspects – beneficence and non maleficence

The principle of beneficence is often seen as the overriding duty in health care. It means the duty to do good, i.e. to act in a way that benefits patients. Non-maleficence requires you not to harm patients intentionally. In treatment decisions at the end of life the dilemma in applying these principles often revolves around what course of action will promote the patient's best interests. In the past best interests was almost always equated with postponing death. But prolonging life may not now automatically be the most ethical approach – not least because modern technology can extend patients' lives beyond the point at which either they desire it or it can benefit them. In short, prolonging life can be harmful. That said it can nonetheless be difficult to see how death can ever be a benefit or in the patient's interests – unless, that is, treatment is so burdensome that continuing it is unquestionably harmful to the patient. Or, to put it another way, in end-of-life decisions the question of how much harm is caused by the treatment needs to be considered, as does the question of whether death itself is always a harm.

This kind of question leads to a discussion of one of the most difficult concepts of all in this context – medical **futility**. Generally the word futility refers to medical treatment that offers no benefit to the patient, i.e. it fails to overcome the patient's medical problem or results in the patient surviving but only leads to a 'useless' life.

The difficulty with the concept of medical futility is that, as Mason *et al.* point out (2002, p. 472), health professionals use the term in four different ways, i.e. for treatment that:

- Is either useless or ineffective
- Fails to offer a minimum quality of life or modicum of medical benefit
- Cannot possibly achieve the patient's goals
- Does not offer a reasonable chance of survival.

But as Mason *et al.* also point out (2002, p. 473), irrespective of the particular approach taken by individual health professionals, in practice futility is typically used as a shorthand way to describe the situation in which a patient demands and health professionals object to the provision of a particular medical treatment on the grounds that it will not provide any medical benefit.

⚷ Keywords

Futility

Medical treatment is generally described as futile in situations where either a) the likelihood of benefiting the patient is so small as to be unrealistic or b) the quality of the benefit to be gained is so minimal that the goals of medicine are not being achieved (Jecker and Schneiderman 1996, p. 170)

> **Key points** ~~Top tips~~
>
> - The principles of beneficence and non-maleficence mean that it is sometimes in patients' interests not to prolong their lives
> - 'Medical futility' is a term health professionals use when they do not consider that treatment will benefit the patient

Legal aspects – a duty not to treat?

In very broad terms one can say that in relation to patients who are dying or incurably ill the legal duty to act in a patient's best interests means a) preventing or retarding a deterioration in their condition and b) the relief of pain and suffering. Several options are therefore lawful, including:

- Withdrawing life-sustaining treatment
- Withholding life-sustaining treatment
- DNAR orders
- Giving pain-killing drugs that may shorten life.

We will look at these options in more detail below. Here we focus on cases in which the concept of futility has been a central issue. As such, they raise the question of whether the legal duty to act in a patient's best interests can (in some circumstances) mean that there is in effect a 'duty not to treat'.

All the cases that have reached the courts in this context have involved either profoundly handicapped babies, patients in a permanent/persistent vegetative state (PVS) or near-PVS, or those who, despite being sensate, are very severely impaired. Consider the cases described in the box below.

Case law – profoundly handicapped babies

Re C [1989]

- **Facts**. A 16-week-old premature baby born with very severe hydrocephalus, C was terminally ill, blind, deaf and suffering from cerebral palsy in all four limbs. Her prognosis was described as 'hopeless'. The court was asked to decide whether life-sustaining treatment such as antibiotics or nasogastric feeding should be given, if, as was inevitable sooner or later, these would be required to keep C alive.
- **Decision**. It was in C's best interests to withhold such treatment on the basis that 'the life which treatment would prolong would be so cruel as to be intolerable'.

continued

Baby J (1990)

- **Facts**. J was born 13 weeks premature (weighing 1.1 kg). He was severely and permanently brain-damaged but neither dying nor near death (his life expectancy was late teens). Five months old when the case came to court he was breathing independently but had been ventilated twice for long periods. The most optimistic prognosis was that he was likely to develop serious spastic quadriplegia, would be blind and deaf, was unlikely ever to speak or develop even limited intellectual abilities but would feel the same pain as a normal infant.

- **Decision**. The doctor's duty to act in J's best interests meant that if he could not continue breathing unaided, there was no legal obligation either to reventilate him or to provide other forms of intensive care.

Re C (1996)

- **Facts**. C was a baby whose condition was described as 'almost a living death' but who could live for months or even up to 2 years. Although C's parents agreed with doctors that ventilation should be discontinued, the case went to court to confirm that withdrawal of treatment was lawful.

- **Decision**. The court had no doubt that it was.

Re C (1998)

- **Facts**. The parents of a baby (who was able to smile and recognise her parents) with spinal muscular atrophy – described as a 'no-chance situation – wanted her to be reventilated.

- **Decision**. The court held that treatment could be withdrawn and resuscitation could be excluded.

Other similar cases involving PVS patients will be discussed below.

Key points ~~Top tips~~

- Case law has established that acting in a patient's best interests can mean that in practice there is in effect a legal 'duty not to treat'

To respect autonomy

Ethical aspects

The principle of respect for autonomy acknowledges that patients have the right to control their her own lives and so can decide when and how to die. This means that competent adults (see Chapter 12 in relation to children) have the right to refuse life-saving treatment (e.g. *Re B* [2002]). But does respecting autonomy go further than this? Does it mean, for example, that a patient can demand assistance in ending his/her life? In this kind of situation the principle of respect for autonomy comes into conflict with other ethical considerations – non-maleficence and beneficence. But notwithstanding the fact that few health professionals now question patients' right to self-determination, it is quite another thing to claim that, as a consequence, they have a moral obligation to help a patient die, i.e. to participate in euthanasia.

Legal aspects

As we saw in Chapter 6 the law strongly supports the principle of respect for autonomy. However, legislation and case law have established beyond doubt that, even though patients may request help to die it is unlawful to assist them. So, for example, if a patient commits suicide by taking an overdose of tablets you have left by the bedside for that purpose, you could be found guilty of assisting suicide (under the Suicide Act 1961). But remember that there is no legal obligation to provide futile treatment. This means that you do not have to provide life-sustaining treatment to patients even if they (or their families) have demanded it (see *A National Health Service Trust* v. *D* [2000]).

> ### Key points   Top tips
>
> - The two key legal and ethical duties owed to terminally and incurably patients are a) to act in their best interests and b) to respect autonomy
> - There is no legal or ethical obligation to provide futile treatment

Important distinctions

In this section we focus on two of the most important distinctions that you need to consider when making end-of-life decisions. The first is the distinction between killing and letting die, and the second is the difference between foreseeing and intending death.

The distinction between killing and letting die

Ethical issues – the acts/omissions doctrine

Keywords

Acts/omissions doctrine
The belief that it is morally worse to actively kill someone than it is to allow them to die by failing to act (to save or preserve their life)

There is a vast literature on the distinction between killing and letting die (also known as the **acts/omissions doctrine**).

Put simply, the doctrine maintains that there is a moral difference between actively killing someone and failing to take action (an omission) that may save or preserve that person's life. Thus it is morally wrong to push someone into a river to their death but we may have no moral duty to leap into the river to save someone who is drowning. In medical situations the acts/omissions distinction means that it is morally worse to kill a patient by, for example, giving a lethal injection (active euthanasia) than it is to allow the patient to die – by, say, withholding life-sustaining treatment (passive euthanasia).

The acts/omissions doctrine is a comforting one for several reasons:

- Most people instinctively feel less responsible and guilty for their omissions than they do for their actions, even if the consequences are the same
- It reflects our assumption (albeit a false one) that 'letting die' is invariably a peaceful process, chosen because it alone best serves the demands of beneficence and non-maleficence (Chadwick and Tadd 1992, p. 168)
- The phrase 'letting die' strongly suggests that the patient is already trying to die so all that we need to do is not stand in their way.

But is there really a moral distinction between giving a lethal injection to a patient in great pain and withdrawing or withholding life-saving treatment from such a patient? After all, in all these three situations the patient will eventually die, albeit sooner following the lethal injection. More importantly, perhaps, is the fact that in all the three situations the behaviour of any health professional involved will be intentional and deliberate. So where does the moral difference lie? And how should the withdrawal and withholding of treatment be classified? Are such 'actions' appropriately described as omissions or do we just describe them like this because it is more psychologically comforting?

One way of justifying the acts/omissions doctrine and distinguishing between killing and letting die is to say that by giving a patient a lethal injection something is made to happen, i.e. death is caused. In contrast, when treatment is withdrawn or withheld it can be said that nature is being allowed to take its course. Thus death is not being made to happen, instead, the omission consists of merely letting something happen, i.e. letting a patient die from the normal progress of his/her disease.

But many commentators reject this distinction on two main grounds. First, it is not always clear whether something is an act or an omission. Second, we are just as responsible for our omissions as we are for our acts. This is because, when faced with a problematic situation, we could take two or more paths. If we choose one path, whether this is to act or to omit to act, both are 'active' choices and so both carry equal moral weight (Hope *et al.* 2003, pp. 164–165).

Legal issues – withdrawal and withholding of treatment

Despite the uncertainty as to whether there is a moral distinction between an act and an omission, the law accepts the distinction unequivocally. In other words there is no doubt that in law there is a fundamental difference between giving a patient a lethal injection (an act) – which is unlawful – and withdrawing or withholding treatment (an omission) – which is lawful.

The leading case that established this legal principle was the famous Bland case (see box below).

Airedale NHS Trust v. *Bland* (1993)

21-year-old Anthony Bland had been crushed in the Hillsborough football stadium disaster. For 3 years he had been in PVS but his brain stem was still functioning. In law, therefore, Anthony was alive. He was able to breath and digest food but could not see, hear, communicate, taste or smell. His bowels were evacuated by enema and a catheter drained his bladder. He was fed through a nasogastric tube and lay in bed with his eyes open and his limbs crooked and taut. He had had repeated infections and had also been operated on for various genitourinary problems. With constant care he could be kept alive for many years but he would never regain consciousness.

The House of Lords decided that discontinuing treatment, including ventilation, nutrition and hydration, was an omission. In other words, stopping life support was simply allowing nature to take its course. Health professionals were not therefore – in law anyway – responsible for his death.

The effect of *Bland* is therefore that:

- Artificial feeding and hydration is medical treatment
- Withdrawing and/or withholding life-sustaining treatment is an omission
- Passive euthanasia is lawful
- Court permission is normally required to withdraw treatment from PVS patients.

Despite the inconsistencies that the Bland case gave rise to (on which see Hendrick 2000, p. 235), the case did provide guidelines as to when life-saving treatment could lawfully be withdrawn in PVC cases – e.g. *Re C* (1996); *Re H* (1997); *NHS Trust A* v. *Mrs M*, *NHS Trust B* v. *Mrs H* (2001). However, the legality of non-treatment decisions in respect of other patients – e.g. those who are not in PVS but who nevertheless have irreversible brain damage – is less clear. It is in these kinds of situation that the distinction between foreseeing and intending death – the so-called double-effect principle – may be relevant.

The distinction between foreseeing and intending a consequence – the double-effect principle

Ethical issues

♂━π Keywords

Double effect

Emphasises the moral difference between what we intend or expect (to relieve pain) and what happens (death is hastened) when we give morphine to a patient in great pain

The ethical principle of **double effect** was developed by Catholic theologians in the Middle Ages to determine in what circumstances an action that has both good and bad consequences is morally right. When, in other words, can you do something that is intended to produce a good result but will also have a harmful effect?

Prescribing pain relief that, in large doses, shortens the life of a terminally ill patient is often used as an example of double effect. Justification for giving the morphine lies in the fact that, although the patient's death is foreseen, it is an indirect result of the treatment and unintended. Or, to put it another way, foreseeing that a bad consequence will occur as a result of doing something is not the same thing as intending that bad consequence.

There are many criticisms of the double-effect principle. Here are some.

It is morally dishonest

The main criticism of double effect is that it is simply not possible to distinguish between a consequence that is intended and one that is foreseen. How, in other words, can you deny that you have 'intended' a consequence that you can foresee is certain, or at least very probable? So if, at the request of a patient who is dying and in unbearable pain, you administer a dose of morphine that you know will shorten his/her life, can you really claim that you did not intend the patient's death but merely foresaw it?

It is no longer appropriate

Current practice in palliative care, in particular sound knowledge of the principles of pain management, proper pain assessment and correct drug administration should help reduce the need to rely on the principle (Johnstone 1999, p. 329). In other words, the assumption here is that pain can be 'controlled'.

It creates an illusion

The illusion (i.e. mistaken belief) created by the double-effect principle is that we do not intend or expect death. The principle has therefore allowed us 'not to confront death, not to take part in it and not to understand the issue of dignity' (Cassell 1996). As Cassell continues:

> in the double-effect doctrine, we must believe that we are not intending death . . . we fool ourselves into thinking that death is an accident or a 'failure', i.e. we were really just trying to treat the pain and it was a failure of medicine that the patient died in the meantime.
>
> Cassell 1996, p. 224

Tschudin makes a similar point (2003, p. 134) when she claims that death is now often seen as 'something like an illness that we prefer to ignore' (in effect the 'worst illness'). And because most illness is dealt with in hospitals, that is where death mostly happens. Death is therefore something that most people see less often (and so are less familiar with than in the past). That explains, at least in part, why it has become 'strange' and consequently 'something to be feared'.

Legal issues

The law first recognised the principle of double effect in the 1957 case of Dr Adams, who was accused of deliberately increasing the dose of opiates used as pain relief in order to end the lives of patients who had left him money in their wills. In summarising the legal position the judge said: '*the doctor is entitled to relieve pain and suffering even if the measures he takes may incidentally shorten life*'. Following this advice the jury acquitted Dr Adams.

The case was controversial – not least because it distorted how the concept of 'intention' had traditionally been interpreted in English criminal law (Hendrick 2000, p. 236). But subsequent case law (e.g. *R* v. *Woollin* [1999]) has confirmed that the administration of drugs that hasten death will be lawful providing the following three tests are satisfied:

- The patient must be already dying
- Prescribing drugs must be the 'right and proper treatment', i.e. accepted as proper by a responsible body of the profession
- The motivation for prescribing drugs must be to relieve pain and suffering (Montgomery 2003, p. 466).

It is lawful to administer drugs that hasten death if:
- The patient is dying
- It is the 'right' treatment
- The intention is to relieve suffering

●━🔑 Keywords

DNAR order
Typically, a direction that in the event of a cardiac arrest neither basic nor advanced life support measures should be started

The 'do not attempt resuscitation' (DNAR) order

The **DNAR order** is usually given by a doctor in an attempt to avoid 'over-treatment' and cardiopulmonary abuses. DNAR orders (sometimes referred to as DNR or NFR orders) are controversial for several reasons:

- **Subjective judgements**. Lack of consultation with patients (and their families) raises the spectre of doctors making ill-thought-out, hasty decisions about lives *they* think are not worth living (Montgomery 2003, p. 474).
- **Age discrimination**. Evidence strongly suggests that DNAR orders are issued more often and more freely in older patients irrespective of the diagnosis and prognosis (Mason *et al.* 2002, p. 565).
- **Inadequate documentation and communication**. Failings in formally recording and communicating DNAR orders – verbal orders are often the most common form of communicating DNAR status – mean that there is often confusion among staff about the procedure (Tschudin 2003, p. 138).

Ethical aspects

'Do not attempt resuscitation' decisions are popularly viewed as medical judgements – about the irreversible nature of a person's disease or illness and their probable poor or hopeless prognosis. But a more accurate interpretation is that they are in fact moral decisions. This is because they are primarily based on moral values – those concerning the 'meaning, sanctity and quality of life' (Johnstone 1999, p. 371). That DNAR decisions involve moral judgements is confirmed by current guidance issued by the NHS, the British Medical Association and the Royal College of Nursing. Briefly, the combined effect of guidance is that a DNAR order should only be made after consultation and consideration of all relevant aspects of the patient's condition. These include:

- The likely benefit from a successful resuscitation if it were achieved

- The patient's known or ascertainable wishes
- The patient's rights including both the right to life and also the right to be free from degrading treatment.

Reflective activity

Identify (and then consider) the moral values in current professional guidance about cardiopulmonary resuscitation (CPR).

Legal aspects

Few cases have reached the courts on the legality of DNAR orders. Nevertheless case law – e.g. *Re J* (1990), *Re R* (1996), *Re C* (1998) – has made it clear that a DNAR order that is supported by unanimous professional opinion and the patient's family will almost always be accepted by the courts as lawful.

Top tips

If you are in any doubt about a DNAR order you should:

- Seek expert advice
- Err on the side of saving life.

You must remember:

- That there must be no blanket policies on DNAR orders
- To assess each patient personally
- Not to base decisions solely on age.

You can find out more about resuscitation policy from:

- NHS Executive, *Resuscitation Policy HSC 2000/028*
- *Resuscitation Council (UK) Decisions Relating to CPR – A joint statement from the BMA and RCN* (2001), available on line at: www.resus.org.uk.

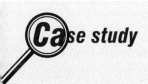
Case study

Basil's advance directive – is it valid?

Basil is 19 and has motor neurone disease. He can only breathe with the help of a ventilator and has very limited ability to communicate, due to the impact of the disease, but is able to do so using eyelid movements. A few days ago he used this method to communicate his wishes, namely that he should be allowed to die 2 weeks after it became impossible to communicate using this last available method. Yesterday he was asked his wishes again while his mother and another carer were present and he confirmed his intention. An anaesthetist and a specialist in palliative care also saw Basil to find out what his wishes were. They received the same answers.

It is expected that Basil will be unable to move his eyelids within the next few weeks.

Case study continued

> ## Reflective activity
>
> 1. What is an advance directive?
> 2. What moral and legal issues does Basil's advance directive raise?

1. Definition of advance directive

Advance directives are also called 'advance statements' or 'living wills'. They are statements made by adults, at a time when they are competent, about how they want to be treated in the future should they become ill and no longer able to make decisions or communicate their wishes. Advance statements can take several different forms. They can be very general – providing a kind of biographical portrait of a person's values and preferences. Or they can be more specific, in which case they typically state in what circumstances (such as when the patient is in a state of irreversible deterioration) life-sustaining treatment should be withheld or withdrawn. Alternatively, an advance directive may operate as an advance refusal of a particular treatment. Advance directives can be oral or written.

2. Moral issues

Ethical issues

Ethical reasons in favour of advance directives include:

- They respect and extend patient autonomy, i.e. they can be considered as a kind of informed consent for the future
- They ensure people have the kinds of end-of-life care they want
- They encourage openness, dialogue and forward planning.

Moral objections to advance directives include:

- Patients may change their minds – as Dworkin notes (1993) a person who drafts a living will and the incompetent who benefits from it are, effectively, different persons and the one need not necessarily be empowered to speak for the other
- Evidence suggest that many patients want in prospect less aggressive treatment than they want when seriously ill – this suggests that people may not be able to imagine future situations sufficiently vividly for their present views to be a good guide to their future wishes
- Treatment decisions are complex, medicine is uncertain, practice is constantly evolving – i.e. advance directives cannot encompass unforeseen possibilities and options.

Legal issues

The facts of this case study are identical to the only reported case of a specific advance decision to die being considered by the court, namely *Re A K* (2001). In accepting that the patient's decision was free and genuine – and therefore legally effective – the judge confirmed that life-support could be withdrawn 2 weeks after A K lost the ability to communicate through using his eyelids.

For an advance refusal to be legally valid (under common law) certain conditions must be met. These are:

Case study continued

- The patient was competent at the time of the refusal
- The refusal was applicable to the current circumstances, i.e. the patient had contemplated the situation that later arose
- The patient was not unduly influenced by anyone, i.e. the decision was an autonomous one
- The patient must have been fully informed of the nature and effect of the treatment that was being refused.

Note: There are proposals in the Mental Capacity Bill 2004 to replace these common law principles with legislation.

Reflective activity

Do you think the advantages of advance directives outweigh their advantages? Do you agree with the court's decision in *Re A K?* Explain your reasons.

The relationship between law and ethics

It is perhaps appropriate that this book should end with a chapter in which law and ethics interact more closely than in any other health-care setting. In the light of this we will summarise some key points.

Ethics

- There is no absolute ethical duty to prolong life at all costs and by all means.
- The principle of double effect maintains that there is a moral difference between intending and foreseeing death.
- The acts and omissions doctrine maintains that there is a moral distinction between killing and letting die.
- Ethical guidelines from professional bodies recognise that, even though there is something special about human life, nevertheless quality-of-life considerations are relevant in making decisions about ending life.

Law

- The courts will never sanction positive steps to end life, i.e. active euthanasia (such as a lethal injection of potassium chloride) is unlawful.
- Competent adult patients (or those who have completed a valid advance directive) have the right to refuse treatment, even if that results in death.
- In some circumstances (i.e. when treatment is not in a patient's best interests) life-prolonging treatment can be withdrawn or withheld – thus legalising passive euthanasia.
- In law there is no difference between withdrawing and withholding treatment; furthermore both are regarded as omissions (i.e. they are considered passive treatment).
- There is no legal obligation to give treatment that is futile.
- The administration of pain-killing drugs may be lawful even if they have the effect of hastening death.
- Although suicide is no longer a crime, assisting suicide is unlawful.

Rapid recap

Check your progress so far by working through each of the following questions.

1. What is the sanctity of life doctrine?
2. What is the principle of double effect?
3. What is a DNAR order?
4. What is an advance directive?

If you have difficulty with more than one of the questions, read through the section again to refresh your understanding before moving on.

References

British Medical Association (2001a) *Withholding and Withdrawing Life Prolonging Medical Treatment*. BMA, London.

British Medical Association (2001b) Decisions relating to cardiopulmonary resuscitation (British Medical Association, UK Resuscitation Council and Royal College of Nursing). *Journal of Medical Ethics* **27** 310–316.

Cassell, E.J. (1996) The sorcerer's broom: medicine's rampant technology. In: *Birth to Death: Science and bioethics* (eds D.C. Thomasma and T. Kushner). Cambridge University Press, Cambridge.

Chadwick, R. and Tadd, W. (1992) *Ethics and Nursing Practice: A case study approach*. Macmillan, Basingstoke.

Cranford, R.E. (1996) Modern technology and the care of the dying. In: *Birth to Death: Science and bioethics* (eds D.C. Thomasma and T. Kushner). Cambridge University Press, Cambridge.

Department of Health (2000) *Resuscitation Policy, HSC 2000/028*. HMSO, London.

Dworkin, G. (1993) *Life's Dominion*. HarperCollins, London.

General Medical Council (2002) *Withholding and Withdrawing Life-prolonging Treatments: Good practice in decision-making*. GMC, London.

Hendrick, J. (2000) *Law and Ethics in Nursing and Health Care*. Stanley Thornes, Cheltenham.

Hope, T., Savulescu, J. and Hendrick, J. (2003) *Medical Ethics and Law: The core curriculum*. Churchill Livingstone, Edinburgh.

Jecker, N.S. and Schneiderman, L.J. (1996) Stopping futile treatment: ethical issues. In: *Birth to Death: Science and bioethics* (eds D.C. Thomasma and T. Kushner). Cambridge University Press, Cambridge.

Johnstone, M.J. (1999) *Bioethics: A nursing perspective*, 3rd edn. Saunders, Marrickville, NSW.

Kennedy, I. and Grubb, A. (2000) *Medical Law*, 3rd edn. Butterworths, London.

Keown, J. (1997) *Euthanasia Examined: Ethical, clinical and legal perspectives*. Cambridge University Press, Cambridge.

Mason, J.K., McCall Smith, R.A. and Laurie, G.T. (2002) *Law and Medical Ethics*, 6th edn. Butterworths, London.

Montgomery, J. (2003) *Health Care Law*. Oxford University Press, Oxford.

Royal College of Paediatrics and Child Health (1997) *Withholding or Withdrawing Life Saving Treatment in Children: A framework for practice*. RCPCH, London.

Singer, P. (1995) *Rethinking Life and Death*. Oxford University Press, Oxford.

Stauch, M., Wheat, K. and Tingle, J. (2002) *Sourcebook on Medical Law*, 2nd edn. Cavendish, London.

Tschudin, V. (2003) *Ethics in Nursing: The caring relationship*, 3rd edn. Butterworth-Heinemann, Edinburgh.

Appendix A

Re T (1997)

Butler-Sloss, Waite and Roch L.JJ.
1996 Sept. 27, 30;
Oct. 24

*Children—Court's inherent jurisdiction—
Medical treatment—Child born with life-
threatening liver defect—Transplant surgery
required to save child's life—Unanimous
medical opinion in favour of treatment—Parents
refusing consent—Reasonableness of refusal—
Whether to be determined solely by clinical
assessment of likely success of treatment—
Whether future treatment to be left to parents*

T. was born in April 1995 with a life-
threatening liver defect and an operation when
he was 3½ weeks old was unsuccessful. The
medical opinion was unanimous that without
undergoing a liver transplantation he would not
live beyond the age of 2½. His parents, who
had gone with him to live and work abroad,
were both health care professionals with
experience in the care of young, sick children.
They did not wish T. to undergo transplant
surgery and refused their consent to an
operation should a suitable liver become
available. The doctors who had treated T. in
England were of the opinion that his parents
were not acting in his best interests and
referred the matter to the relevant local
authority, which applied under section 100(3)
of the Children Act 1989 for the court to
exercise its inherent wardship jurisdiction. The
judge held that the mother's refusal to accept
the unanimous advice of the doctors and her
refusal to consent to the operation was not the

conduct of a reasonable parent and he ordered
that T. be returned to the jurisdiction within 21
days to be assessed for transplant surgery.

On appeal by the mother:—

Held, allowing the appeal, that when an
application was made to the court under its
inherent jurisdiction the welfare of the child
was the paramount consideration and,
although a parent's consent or refusal of
consent was an important consideration to
weigh in the balancing exercise, it was for the
court to decide the matter and in so doing it
might overrule the decision of a reasonable
parent; that the judge had erred in not
weighing in the balance reasons against the
treatment which might be held by a reasonable
parent on much broader grounds than that of
clinical assessment of the likely success of the
proposed treatment, and his decision therefore
could not stand; that, taking into account the
unusual facts, the significance of the close
attachment between the mother and T. and the
practical difficulties inherent in implementing
an order for T.'s return and treatment, it was in
his best interests to require his future
treatment to be left in the hands of his parents;
and that, accordingly, the judge's order would
be set aside (post, pp. 250D-H, 251H-252B,
253A-C, C-D, 254B-D, 256D-E, 257A-B).

*In re J. (A Minor) (Wardship: Medical
Treatment)* [1991] Fam. 33, C.A. and *In re Z
(A Minor) (Identification: Restrictions on
Publication)* [1997] Fam. 1, C.A. applied.

Decision of Connell J. reversed.

The following cases are referred to in the judgments:

B. *(A Minor) (Wardship: Medical Treatment), In re* [1981] 1 W.L.R. 1421; [1990] 3 All ER. 927, C.A.

B. *(A Minor) (Wardship: Sterilisation), In re* [1988] AC. 199; [1987] 2 W.L.R. 1213; [1987] 2 All E.R. 206, H.L.(E.)

G. *v. G. (Minors: Custody Appeal)* [1985] 1 W.L.R. 647; [1985] 2 All E.R. 225, H.L.(E)

J. *(A Minor) (Wardship: Medical Treatment), In re* [1991] Fam. 33; [1991] 2 W.L.R. 140; [1990] 3 All E.R. 930, C.A.

W. *(A Minor) (Medical Treatment: Court's Jurisdiction), In re* [1993] Fam. 64; [1992] 3 W.L.R. 758; [1992] 4 All E.R. 627, C.A.

Z *(A Minor) (Identification: Restrictions on Publication), In re* [1997] Fam. 1; [1996] 2 W.L.R. 88; [1995] 4 All E.R. 961, C.A.

The following additional cases were cited in argument:

Airedale N.H.S. Trust v. Bland [1993] A.C. 789; [1993] 2 W.L.R. 316; [1993] 1 All E.R. 821, H.L.(E.)

D. *(A Minor) (Wardship: Sterilisation), In re* [1976] Fam. 185; [1976] 2 W.L.R. 279; [1976] 1 All E.R. 326

Frenchay Healthcare National Health Service Trust v. S. [1994] 1 W.L.R. 601; [1994] 2 All E.R. 403, C.A.

Gillick v. West Norfolk and Wisbech Area Health Authority [1986] A.C. 112; [1985] 3 W.L.R. 830; [1985] 3 All E.R. 402, H.L.(E.)

Harben v. Harben [1957] 1 W.L.R. 261; [1957] 1 All E.R. 379

Hope v. Hope (1854) 4 De G.M. & G. 328

J. *v. C.* [1970] A.C. 668; [1969] 2 W.L.R. 540; [1969] 1 All E.R. 788, H.L.(E.)

Liddell's Settlement Trusts, In re [1936] Ch. 365; [1936] 1 All E.R. 239, C.A.

P. *(A Minor), In re* [1986] 1 F.L.R. 272

P. *(G.E.) (An Infant), In re* [1965] Ch. 568; [1965] 2 W.L.R. 1; [1964] 3 All E.R. 977, C.A.

Rex v. Sandbach Justices, Ex parte Smith [1951] 1 K.B. 62; [1950] 2 All E.R. 781, D.C.

Sidaway v. Board of Governors of the Bethlem Royal Hospital and the Maudsley Hospital [1985] A.C. 871; [1985] 2 W.L.R. 480; [1985] 1 All E.R. 643, H.L.(E.)

W. *(A Minor) (Contact), In re* [1994] 2 F.L.R. 441, C.A.

APPEAL from Connell J.

T., born in 1995, had a liver defect and the unanimous medical opinion was that without an organ transplant he would not live beyond the age of $2^1/_2$. His parents, who had gone with T. to live and work overseas, refused to give their consent to transplant surgery. The local authority, having been granted leave to make an application to the court for it to exercise its inherent jurisdiction and the Official Solicitor being appointed T.'s guardian ad litem, contended that the parents' refusal was in the circumstances not reasonable and that it was in T.'s best interests to undergo a liver transplantation. On 17 September 1996 the judge ordered the mother to return T. to the jurisdiction within 21 days for the purposes of assessment for liver transplantation and to undergo such surgery as might be advised by those medically responsible for him. He granted the mother leave to appeal.

By a notice of appeal dated September 1996 the mother appealed on grounds that (1) the judge was wrong in finding the mother's refusal to consent unreasonable when (a) the medical team to whom the judge envisaged T. being referred for surgery considered the mother's view reasonable; (b) T.'s parents as neonatal nurses had unique experience in the care of severely ill children; (c) the risks and inevitable consequences of the procedure were such that it was obviously considered necessary by one of the doctors to warn the parents of them so as to enable them to take them into account in deciding whether to consent; (d) there was unchallenged evidence that a responsible medical practice existed of respecting parents' wishes and that the parents were informed by those recommending a transplant that such was the practice; (e) the requirement in law that parental consent to the procedure be obtained before it could be lawfully performed had the consequence of obliging the parents to carry out the very exercise of judgment in the interest of T. that the parents had performed; that decision should not be made on medical grounds alone; (f) doctors in the country where the parents were living were prepared to respect the mother's views; (g) the mother was loving and caring and was acting in good faith in what she believed to be the best interests of T. and therefore she should be regarded as the best judge of his best interests; and (h) contrary to the judge's findings, the mother came to her view before she could have been influenced by any perceived improvement in T.'s condition; (2) if the mother's refusal of consent was not unreasonable, the judge was wrong to proceed to decide for himself what were the best interests of T.; (3) the judge was wrong to make an order in effect requiring T. to undergo major surgery which would inevitably require devoted post-operative care to be provided by the mother throughout the rest of his life, when the mother had decided in good faith that such surgery was not in his best interests; (4) the court was wrong to exercise its inherent jurisdiction to make an order directing the mother to return T. to the jurisdiction and to permit the transplant despite her lack of consent, when (a) T. and both parents were lawfully then and for the foreseeable future resident out of the jurisdiction; (b) there was no evidence or finding by the court that the medical facilities

available to T. locally were inadequate; (c) none of the doctors who gave evidence to the court owed any current or continuing duty of care to T., and (d) there was evidence that the local authorities would not seek to procure a transplant without parental consent; (5) the judge was wrong to make an order which was plainly incapable of working as he envisaged since (a) he accepted that there was no basis for a working relationship between the mother and the medical team concerned and that it was not in T.'s best interest for any transplant to be carried out in their hospital; (b) if the mother complied with the order by presenting T. to the hospital specified in the judge's order, there was evidence that the team there would not perform a transplant; (c) if she complied with the order by presenting T. to an alternative hospital (the only other centre in the jurisdiction) and the team there were prepared to perform the procedure without her consent (as to which there was no firm evidence) that would lead to a breakdown in the working relationship with the mother and therefore give rise to the same impasse reached at the first-mentioned hospital; (d) if transplant surgery were to be performed there would be a continuing need for specialised care, the strong possibility of further surgery and continuing court supervision, in the absence of parental consent; (e) in the premises the order was unworkable unless the mother were to consent to the procedure, in which case the order would be unnecessary, and (f) in such circumstances it was wrong in principle to make an order under the inherent jurisdiction in a mere attempt to persuade a parent to change his or her mind.

The facts are stated in the judgment of Butler-Sloss L.J.

> *Robert Francis Q.C.* and *Andrew Hockton* for the mother.
>
> *David Harris Q.C.* and *Yvonne Coppel* for the local authority.

Gordon Murdoch Q.C. and *Huw Lloyd* for the guardian ad litem.

Cur. adv. vult.

24 October. The following judgments were handed down.

BUTLER-SLOSS L.J. T. was born on 10 April 1995 suffering from biliary atresia, a life-threatening liver defect. The unanimous medical prognosis is that he will not live beyond the age of 2 to $2^{1}/_{2}$ without a liver transplantation. It is equally the unanimous clinical opinion of the consultants that it is in his interests to undergo the operation when a donor liver becomes available. The parents, who were trained as health care professionals and are both experienced in the care of young sick children, do not wish the operation to take place. The main issue before the judge and on appeal before this court is whether the court should overrule the decision of the parents and consent to the operation. It arises as a specific issue in respect of which the court is asked to exercise its inherent jurisdiction.

The background to this tragic and deeply worrying case is as follows. The parents are not married but have a stable relationship. They decided to apply for jobs in a distant Commonwealth country ("country AB"). The father went to country AB in September 1995 while T. and his mother remained in England with her family. In February 1996 the mother took T. to visit his father but returned with him in April to England. They went back to country AB in June 1996 and remain there now. The mother gave evidence to Connell J. in the proceedings, the subject of this appeal, by video link.

Once T.'s liver defect was diagnosed the medical advice at the local hospital was for him to undergo an operation called "Kasai" with the hope that this would improve his condition. The parents agreed and he underwent the operation at the age of $3^{1}/_{2}$ weeks but the outcome was unsuccessful. The mother's view of the proposed liver transplantation operation has been much influenced by the circumstances of the Kasai operation and the pain and distress caused to the baby both by it and by the consequential treatment. She and the father came to the conclusion, having sought medical advice, that if the Kasai operation proved unsuccessful they would not wish their baby to undergo major transplant surgery.

The mother and child were then referred to one of the few hospitals which carry out liver transplantation operations ("hospital X"). She met the consultant paediatrician, Dr. A., and her team and between September and November 1995 T. was assessed for his suitability and found to be suitable to have the transplantation operation. The mother was supplied with printed information about the operation called *Liver Transplantation: An Introduction: Fact Sheet No. 10*, published by the Children's Liver Disease Foundation. It said that it was:

"one of the most major forms of surgery. It is more complicated than other transplant operations on other organs and is only considered when other forms of treatment no longer maintain a good quality of life. . . . The team will discuss the results of the tests with the parents and tell them whether their child or baby is a suitable candidate for transplant. It is a very big decision to make on the part of the family and every assistance will be given to help to make the decision. If the family choose not to proceed with the transplantation once they are acquainted with the facts, the decision is respected. The child and family will continue to receive the necessary medical and nursing care to give him/her the best quality of life."

The mother did not consent to the carrying out of the operation. Dr. A. made it clear to the mother that it was in the best interests of T. that the operation be carried out and could not accept the mother's reasons for refusing to consent. Inevitably the relationship between Dr. A. and the mother became strained. Dr. A. told the mother that the hospital would seek legal advice if the mother did not consent. The mother obtained a second opinion from a consultant paediatrician, Dr. P., at hospital Y, another centre of liver transplant operations. Dr. P. set out his conclusions in a letter dated 6 December 1995 which was sent to the mother's general practitioner. Despite referring to adverse factors, which are no longer of significance in the light of later evidence, Dr. P. wrote:

"I would consider an excellent result of transplantation to be many years of life with normal growth with no treatment necessary other than irnmuno-suppression, and there is certainly a good chance that such an outcome could be achieved."

He and his team strongly urged the mother to consent to the offer of transplantation at hospital X, but said that, if she and the father after further consideration did not consent, that decision should be respected.

T. was placed on the urgent transplant list at hospital X. The mother then took him to country AB against the advice of Dr. A. Whilst there T. was under the care of a consultant paediatrician, but there are no facilities for a liver transplant operation in that country. A suitable liver became available at hospital X while the mother was abroad with the baby, but the hospital was unable to get in touch with the mother and the opportunity was lost. Dr. A.'s team formed the view that the mother was not acting in the best interests of T. and they took legal advice. The matter was referred to the local authority of the mother's area who involved their child protection team. The police

in country AB were informed and visited the mother. The child was found to be well and happy. They concluded, supported by the local social services, that no action was needed. On the return of the mother and T. to England in April they were again referred to hospital Y and Dr. P. was asked to take over the care of T. The mother continued to oppose the carrying out of the operation. Dr. P. discussed the matter with her at length on several occasions. He and his team formed the view that she was a loving and devoted mother, and, from her professional background, an unusually well-informed parent. They concluded that her reluctance to submit her son to the operation was founded in love and care for him. She was to the best of her ability discharging her duty of trust to her child and her decision should be respected.

The mother then returned to country AB with T. and on 17 July 1996 the local authority sought the leave of the court to commence proceedings under the provisions of section 100(3) of the Children Act 1989. Its application was granted by Hollis J. on 27 August 1996. The Official Solicitor was appointed guardian ad litem of the child and he instructed a consultant surgeon, Mr. R., from hospital Z.

At the substantive hearing of the application of the local authority, Connell J. heard evidence from Dr. P., Mr. R. and Dr. A., all distinguished consultants in this specialist field. Dr. P. accepted the opinion of Mr. R. as to the likely success of the transplant operation. In their reports and in their oral evidence the three doctors were unanimous that the prospects of success were good and that this operation was in the best interests of the child. Dr. A. and her team were prepared to carry out the operation without the consent of the mother if the court gave consent. The judge felt that the breakdown in the relationship between the mother and the team of Dr. A. made hospital X unsuitable in the best interests of T. Dr. P. and his team, while strongly recommending the operation, would wish to respect the decision of the mother and would not be prepared to perform the operation without her consent. Mr. R. was prepared to carry out the operation but could not answer for his team in the event that the mother did not consent.

The local authority in its originating summons sought the answers to three specific questions: whether it was in the best interests of T. (i) to undergo surgery for a liver transplantation, (ii) for permission to be granted to perform the surgery notwithstanding the refusal of the mother to consent, and (iii) for the child to be returned to the jurisdiction for the purpose of such surgery. It was neutral before the judge and the proposed surgery was strongly advocated by T.'s guardian ad litem.

Connell J., on 17 September 1996, in a careful, comprehensive and sensitive judgment reviewed the reasons for the mother's refusal to consent and said:

"In my judgment it has proved impossible for this mother to accept the main burden of the advice of the doctors, which is to the effect that if T. does not undergo a transplant he will die within the next 12 to 18 months. Clinging to her own ability to provide expert care for this little boy and observing his apparent improvement in health, I am satisfied that she has not as yet really been able to face up to the clear and unanimous conclusion of the doctors that transplantation would be in his best interests. Whilst I can understand her difficulties, I conclude that her refusal to accept the unanimous advice of the doctors is not the conduct of a reasonable parent."

He answered the three questions posed by the local authority in the affirmative and directed the return of the mother with T. to the jurisdiction within 21 days in order to undergo the surgery for liver transplantation. He directed that the child be presented to hospital Y or hospital Z for assessment for transplantation. He concluded:

"In reaching a decision in cases such as this case the court is required to balance a number of factors. I have considered that quality of life which is likely to be available to the little boy post transplantation, and I have considered the pain and suffering which is likely to be undergone either with or without transplantation. There is of course a strong presumption in favour of preserving life, but this is not an absolute rule. It is clear that T. will die without transplantation, that treatment is available to him, and it is recommended as in his best interests by the three doctors who gave evidence to the court. In all the circumstances, and in the light of all the evidence, I reach the clear conclusion that it is appropriate to make orders as sought."

He expressed the hope that the mother might change her mind and consent to the operation. He gave leave to appeal.

On the appeal Mr. Francis, for the mother, informed us that the mother has not changed her mind and that she continued to be supported in her views by the father. He challenged the judge's conclusion that the mother's refusal to consent was unreasonable. He relied heavily upon the opinion of Dr. P. that he and his team respected the mother's decision and would not seek to go behind it and their view of the enormous importance of the total co-operation of the mother to the operation and the consequential treatment. In most medical situations there was more than one answer. The doctors' view was based upon clinical grounds, but where the welfare of a child required a family decision that decision if reasonable ought to be respected and the inherent jurisdiction of the court ought not to be exercised to overrule it. The more borderline the decision the more weight should be given to the parents' view. He stressed the possibility of further operations and further treatment and the effect upon the mother and upon the child. The choice was to allow the child a short life where he was well and happy for most of the time and would be likely to die peacefully or to cause him to undergo major invasive surgery with a good success rate but all the risks, discomfort and distress for a young child and a lifetime of drugs and the possibility of further invasive surgery and other treatment. The consequence of the decision was to commit the mother to a lifetime of care of the child with the requirement of total commitment to the treatment. The importance of the element of morale was not to be underestimated. The mother would find it very difficult to support the treatment, despite her specialist training and her devotion to the child. Since transplant operations have only been performed for 14 years on children, the statistics were inadequate as a guide for the future. He drew a distinction between extending life and allowing a child to die prematurely. The mother's decision was within that band of reasonable decisions with which the court should not interfere and coerce the mother.

Mr. Harris for the local authority and Mr. Murdoch for the Official Solicitor as guardian ad litem of T. strongly supported the decision of the judge that the transplant operation was in the best interests of T. They argued that the judge was entitled to come to the conclusion that the mother's refusal of consent was unreasonable in the light of unanimous medical opinion that this was the accepted treatment and the surgery gave the child a good chance of an extended and a reasonable quality of life. The test was welfare of the child

and not the reasonableness of the parent. The view of the parents was only one factor in the welfare test. We were reminded of the enormous strides which continue to be made in medical knowledge and techniques which supported the good prospects of success for the child. There was no reason to suppose that, if the operation was carried out, this mother with her special abilities would not respond to the needs of the child and care for him with devotion and competence. Mr. Murdoch stressed that the practical difficulties were not insuperable and should be met if or when they arose.

I turn to consider previous decisions which set out the principles to be followed in an application such as this which invokes the inherent jurisdiction of the High Court. In recent years the medical profession and local authorities have increasingly sought declarations or directions from the High Court in difficult medical issues which involve ethical as well as medical considerations, for instance, abortion or sterilisation. Applications have also been made to the court in a number of cases which might affect the continued life of the child or adult. In the past applications in respect of children were made within the ambit of wardship. It is, however, clear that wardship is a mechanism within which to seek the decision of the High Court and it is not necessary to make the child a ward in order to invoke the inherent jurisdiction of the court: see Sir Thomas Bingham M.R. in *In re Z (A Minor) (Identification: Restrictions on Publication)* [1997] Fam. 1, 32.

A line of cases from 1981 has, in my judgment, clearly established the approach of the court to these most difficult and anxious questions. In *In re B. (A Minor) (Wardship: Medical Treatment)* [1981] 1 W.L.R. 1421 the child was born suffering from Down's syndrome and from an intestinal blockage which required to be relieved by an operation if she were not to die within a few days. The surgeon respected the wishes of the parents not to consent to the operation and decided not to operate. The judge took the same view. This court allowed the appeal and held that the question for the court was whether it was in the best interests of the child that she should have the operation and not whether the wishes of the parents should be respected. In that case the evidence disclosed that if the operation was performed the child would live the normal span of life of a mongol.

The House of Lords in *In re B. (A Minor) (Wardship: Sterilisation)* [1988] A.C. 199 held that a court exercising wardship jurisdiction, when reaching a decision on an application to authorise an operation for sterilisation of the ward, was concerned with only one primary and paramount consideration, the welfare of the child.

This court in *In re J. (A Minor) (Wardship: Medical Treatment)* [1991] Fam. 33 considered the future medical management of a severely brain-damaged premature baby with a considerably shortened life expectancy. Lord Donaldson of Lymington M.R. said, at p. 41:

"it is sensible to define the relationship between the court, the doctors, the child and its parents. The doctors owe the child a duty to care for it in accordance with good medical practice recognised as appropriate by a competent body of professional opinion: see *Bolam v. Friern Hospital Management Committee* [1957] 1 W.L.R. 582. This duty is, however, subject to the qualification that, if time permits, they must obtain the consent of the parents before undertaking serious invasive treatment. The parents owe the child a duty to give or to withhold consent in the best interests of the child and without regard to their own interests. The court when exercising the parens patriae

jurisdiction takes over the rights and duties of the parents, although this is not to say that the parents will be excluded from the decision-making process. Nevertheless in the end the responsibility for the decision whether to give or to withhold consent is that of the court alone."

He concluded, at pp. 46–47:

"*In re B. (A Minor) (Wardship: Medical Treatment)* [1981] 1 W.L.R. 1421 seems to me to come very near to being a binding authority for the proposition that there is a balancing exercise to be performed in assessing the course to be adopted in the best interests of the child. Even if it is not, I have no doubt that this should be and is the law. This brings me face to face with the problem of formulating the critical equation. In truth it cannot be done with mathematical or any precision. There is without doubt a very strong presumption in favour of a course of action which will prolong life, but, even excepting the 'cabbage' case to which special considerations may well apply, it is not irrebuttable. As this court recognised in *In re B.*, account has to be taken of the pain and suffering and quality of life which the child will experience if life is prolonged. Account has also to be taken of the pain and suffering involved in the proposed treatment itself . . . . in the end there will be cases in which the answer must be that it is not in the interests of the child to subject it to treatment which will cause increased suffering and produce no commensurate benefit, giving the fullest possible weight to the child's, and mankind's, desire to survive."

In *In re Z (A Minor) (Identification: Restrictions on Publication)* [1997] Fam. 1 the main issue was whether the child was to be identified and allowed to participate in a television film about her upbringing. The question whether the courts should intervene in a situation where a mother exercised her parental responsibilities bona fide and reasonably was directly before this court. Sir Thomas Bingham M.R. said, at pp. 32–33:

> "I would for my part accept without reservation that the decision of a devoted and responsible parent should be treated with respect. It should certainly not be disregarded or lightly set aside. But the role of the court is to exercise an independent and objective judgment. If that judgment is in accord with that of the devoted and responsible parent, well and good. If it is not, then it is the duty of the court, after giving due weight to the view of the devoted and responsible parent, to give effect to its own judgment. That is what it is there for. Its judgment may of course be wrong. So may that of the parent. But once the jurisdiction of the court is invoked its clear duty is to reach and express the best judgment it can."

From the decisions to which I have referred which bind this court it is clear that when an application under the inherent jurisdiction is made to the court the welfare of the child is the paramount consideration. The consent or refusal of consent of the parents is an important consideration to weigh in the balancing exercise to be carried out by the judge. In that context the extent to which the court will have regard to the view of the parent will depend upon the court's assessment of that view. But, as Sir Thomas Bingham M.R. said in *In re Z*, the court decides and in doing so may overrule the decision of a reasonable parent.

Applying those principles, to the present appeal, the first argument of Mr. Francis that the court should not interfere with the reasonable decision of a parent is not one that we are able to entertain even if we wished to do so. His suggestion that the decision of this mother came within that band of reasonable decisions within which a court would not interfere would import into this jurisdiction the test applied in adoption to the refusal of a parent to consent to adoption. It is wholly inapposite to the welfare test and is incompatible with the decision in *In re Z*.

In my view, however, the judge erred in his approach to the issue before the court. He accepted the unchallenged clinical opinion of the three consultants and assessed the reasonableness of the mother's decision against that medical opinion. Having held that the mother was unreasonable he accepted that the liver transplant would be likely to prolong the life of T. and in the absence of any reasonable argument to the contrary he came to the clear conclusion that he should consent to the operation. Since he had already decided the mother's approach was unreasonable he did not weigh in the balance reasons against the treatment which might be held by a reasonable parent on much broader grounds than the clinical assessment of the likely success of the proposed treatment. Some of the objections of the mother, such as the difficulties of the operation itself, turned out, from the evidence of Mr. R., to be less important than the mother believed. Underlying those less important objections by the mother was a deep-seated concern of the mother as to the benefits to her son of the major invasive surgery and post-operative treatment, the dangers of failure long term as well as short term, the possibility of the need for further transplants, the likely length of life, and the effect upon her son of all these concerns. The judge did not assess the relevance or the weight of such considerations in his final balancing exercise. In particular he did not consider at that stage the evidence of

Dr. P. and his strong reservations to the effect of coercing, as Dr. P. put it, this mother into playing the crucial and irreplaceable part in the aftermath of major invasive surgery not just during the post-operative treatment of an 18-month-old baby but also throughout the childhood of her son. She would inevitably be the primary carer (no one suggested that this baby should be taken into care) and would be expected to care for him for many years through surgery and continuing treatment while she, on her present view, believed that this course was not right for her son. The total commitment of the caring parent, in Dr. P.'s view, was essential to the success of the treatment. Mr. Harris suggested to us that Dr. P.'s evidence supporting the mother's approach lacked logic and was woolly. That suggestion is, in my view, to underestimate the experience of a distinguished consultant paediatrician in a specialist and still experimental area of medicine. Moreover his evidence was supported by the advice given to parents by hospital X in its *Fact Sheet No. 10.*

I have well in mind the important principles set out by the House of Lords in *G. v. G. (Minors: Custody Appeal)* [1985] 1 W.L.R. 647 and that this most experienced judge saw the witnesses and in particular the mother. If the decision in this case was a matter of assessing the clinical opinions of the doctors, the judge was clearly right to prefer their views to the mother's, who could not be as well qualified to give an opinion. But this matter has to be looked at more broadly. The mother certainly told the judge that she recognised her son had only a short time to live if no operation was performed. She was focusing, it seems to me, on the present peaceful life of the child who had the chance to spend the rest of his short life without the pain, stress and upset of intrusive surgery against the future with the operation and treatment taking place. That is an alternative point of view to that to which the

judge came and, with some hesitation, I doubt that he was right to deem the mother to be unreasonable in her assessment of the broader perspective of whether this operation should be carried out. But in any event the reasonableness of the mother was not the primary issue. This mother and this child are one for the purpose of this unusual case and the decision of the court to consent to the operation jointly affects the mother and son and it also affects the father. The welfare of this child depends upon his mother. The practical considerations of her ability to cope with supporting the child in the face of her belief that this course is not right for him, the requirement to return probably for a long period to this country, either to leave the father behind and lose his support or to require him to give up his present job and seek one in England, were not put by the judge into the balance when he made his decision.

Despite the conclusion of the judge which I have set out above, I do not believe that he put into the balance these broader considerations. Consequently in my view his exercise of discretion was flawed and I am satisfied that his decision cannot stand.

It falls therefore for this court to make the decision whether to consent to the operation and require the return of the child to the jurisdiction. I agree with Mr. Murdoch that this court ought not to make a decision on so difficult and delicate an issue mainly on the problems of ordering the return of the child when he is out of the jurisdiction, or in ignorance of whether hospital Z would in fact carry out the operation if the mother continued in her refusal to consent. But they are none the less relevant considerations which, in my judgment, have to be taken into account in the balancing exercise, although they are not determinative. More important than those considerations is to my mind the evidence of Dr. P. and the emphasis he placed throughout his evidence upon the requirements both of the consent of the parents and of a total commitment by the caring parent to the proposed treatment. He foresaw grave difficulties in carrying out the operation and the treatment without that wholehearted support of the mother.

In *In re W. (A Minor) (Medical Treatment: Court's Jurisdiction)* [1993] Fam. 64, 76, a case about the medical treatment of a girl of 16 suffering from anorexia nervosa, Lord Donaldson of Lymington M.R. said that there were two purposes to seeking consent, clinical and legal:

> "The clinical purpose stems from the fact that in many instances the co-operation of the patient and the patient's faith or at least confidence in the [efficacy] of the treatment is a major factor contributing to the treatment's success."

That passage applies, in my judgment, with equal force to the need for the confidence in and the commitment to the proposed treatment by the principal carer on the unusual facts of this case. Unlike the intestinal obstruction of the Down's syndrome baby which could be cured by a simple operation, T.'s problems require complicated surgery and many years of special care from the mother.

The reservations of Dr. P., to which he held despite concessions he made in his evidence, remain of great significance and importance. His view that the decision of a loving, caring mother should be respected, ought to be given great weight and are reinforced by *Fact Sheet No. 10* provided by hospital X. The alternative of the court giving the consent and passing back the responsibility for the parental care to the mother and expecting her to provide the commitment to the child after the operation is carried out in the face of her opposition is in itself fraught with danger for the child. She will have to comply with the court order; return to

this country and present the child to one of the hospitals. She will have to arrange to remain in this country for the foreseeable future. Will the father stay in country AB and work or come with her to England, giving up his job and having to seek another job? If he does not come she will have to manage unaided. How will the mother cope? Can her professionalism overcome her view that her son should not be subjected to this distressing procedure? Will she break down? How will the child be affected by the conflict with which the mother may have to cope? What happens if the treatment is partially successful and another transplant is needed? The mother may not wish to consent to the further surgery. Is the court to be asked again for consent to the next operation?

The welfare of the child is the paramount consideration and I recognise the "very strong presumption in favour of a course of action which will prolong life" and the inevitable consequences for the child of not giving consent. But to prolong life, as Lord Donaldson of Lymington M.R. recognised in *In re J. (A Minor) (Wardship: Medical Treatment)* [1991] Fam. 33 in somewhat different circumstances, is not the sole objective of the court and to require it at the expense of other considerations may not be in a child's best interests. I would stress that, on the most unusual facts of this case with the enormous significance of the close attachment between the mother and baby, the court is not concerned with the reasonableness of the mother's refusal to consent but with the consequences of that refusal and whether it is in the best interests of T. for this court in effect to direct the mother to take on this total commitment where she does not agree with the course proposed. The effect of the evidence of Dr. P. respecting the mother's decision and the prospect of forcing the devoted mother of this young baby to the consequences of this major invasive surgery lead me to the conclusion, after much anxious deliberation, that it is not in the best interests of this child to give consent and require him to return to England for the purpose of undergoing liver transplantation. I believe that the best interests of this child require that his future treatment should be left in the hands of his devoted parents. Once the pressure of this litigation is over it may be the parents will reconsider whether they should remain in country AB or should return to this country and attend at hospital Y with a view to a further assessment for the purpose of carrying out the operation. That, however, will be a matter for them and not for this court.

I would allow this appeal and would answer the three questions posed in the originating summons in the negative and would set aside the orders of the judge.

WAITE L.J. I agree. The law's insistence that the welfare of a child shall be paramount is easily stated and universally applauded, but the present case illustrates, poignantly and dramatically, the difficulties that are encountered when trying to put it into practice. Throughout his clear and able judgment, the judge demonstrated his appreciation of the dilemma to which the case gives rise. Loving and devoted parents have taken, after anxious consideration, a decision to withhold consent to operative transplant treatment. Although it is relatively novel treatment, still unavailable in many countries, doctors of the highest expertise have unanimously recommended it for this child on clinical grounds, taking the view that it involves a relatively minor level of risk which they regard as well worth taking in the child's long-term interests (which in this instance include an extension of life itself). The parents' opposition is partly instinctive and, being based on their own awareness of the procedures involved, partly practical. It has sufficient cogency to have led one of the principal medical experts in the field of this

operation to say that his team would decline to operate without the mother's committed support.

What is the court to do in such a situation? It is not an occasion—even in an age preoccupied with "rights"—to talk of the rights of a child, or the rights of a parent, or the rights of the court. The cases cited by Butler-Sloss L.J. are uncompromising in their assertion that the sole yardstick must be the need to give effect to the demands of paramountcy for the welfare of the child. They establish that there are bound to be occasions when such paramountcy will compel the court, acting as a judicial parent, to substitute the judge's own views as to the claims of child welfare over those of natural parents—even in a case where the views of the latter are supported by qualities of devotion, commitment, love and reason. The judge, after anxious consideration, reached the conclusion that this case provides such an occasion. Was he right to do so? Of course, if his decision was founded on a correct application of legal principle, it is unassailable, however tempted individual members of an appellate court might be to substitute a judgment of our own. These decisions, not least because they are so difficult and finely balanced, are best left to the discretion of the experienced judges who have the task, often a lonely and worrying one, of weighing the numerous delicate elements—including the view taken of the parties and witnesses—which enable a cumulative picture to be formed of the demands of welfare in a particular case, and taking the momentous decision which the child patient cannot take for himself.

In this instance, however, in agreement with Butler-Sloss L.J., I consider that the judge was betrayed into an error of law by his concern with the need to form a judgment about the reasonableness of the mother's approach. An appraisal of parental reasonableness may be appropriate in other areas of family law (in adoption, for example, where it is enjoined by statute) but when it comes to an assessment of the demands of the child patient's welfare, the starting point—and the finishing point too—must always be the judge's own independent assessment of the balance of advantage or disadvantage of the particular medical step under consideration. In striking that balance, the judge will of course take into account as a relevant, often highly relevant, factor the attitude taken by a natural parent, and that may require examination of his or her motives. But the result of such an inquiry must never be allowed to prove determinative. It is a mistake to view the issue as one in which the clinical advice of doctors is placed in one scale and the reasonableness of the parent's view in the other. Had the judge viewed the evidence more broadly from the standpoint of his own perception of the child's welfare when appraised in all its aspects, he would have |been bound, in my view, to take significant account of other elements in the case. Those include the parents' ties in country AB, and, crucially, the evidence of Dr. P. No one disputes that in the aftermath of the operation the child would remain in the primary care of the mother. Dr. P. maintained a very clear view that—even assuming that the operation proved wholly successful in surgical terms—the child's subsequent development could be injuriously affected if his day-to-day care depended upon the commitment of a mother who had suffered the turmoil of having her child being compelled against her will to undergo, as a result of a coercive order from the court, a major operation against which her own medical and maternal judgment wholeheartedly rebelled.

All these cases depend on their own facts and render generalisations—tempting though they may be to the legal or social analyst—wholly out of place. It can only be said safely

that there is a scale, at one end of which lies the clear case where parental opposition to medical intervention is prompted by scruple or dogma of a kind which is patently irreconcilable with principles of child health and welfare widely accepted by the generality of mankind; and that at the other end lie highly problematic cases where there is genuine scope for a difference of view between parent and judge. In both situations it is the duty of the judge to allow the court's own opinion to prevail in the perceived paramount interests of the child concerned, but in cases at the latter end of the scale, there must be a likelihood (though never of course a certainty) that the greater the scope for genuine debate between one view and another the stronger will be the inclination of the court to be influenced by a reflection that in the last analysis the best interests of every child include an expectation that difficult decisions affecting the length and quality of its life will be taken for it by the parent to whom its care has been entrusted by nature.

I, too, would allow this appeal and substitute the order proposed by Butler-Sloss L.J.

ROCH L.J. This is a desperately difficult case. The medical evidence was, as the judge stressed, unanimous on the prognosis for this child if he did not receive a transplanted liver: he will die in a matter of months. The doctors went further and said that, despite those matters which mean that the child is not the ideal recipient of a liver transplant, he was nevertheless a good candidate with good prospects for a favourable outcome.

On the other hand, no one suggests that the child's parents are not responsible parents who are devoted to this child or that they have not spent much time and thought in reaching their decision that their son should not undergo a liver transplant and the treatment that will inevitably follow such an operation. The evidence indicated that because of their training and experience they are "uniquely well qualified" to make a decision. In my view, it cannot be said on the evidence that was before the judge that their decision was unreasoned.

What principles should apply to a case such as this? The paramount principle is that the court must make the decision which it considers to be in the best interests of the child. In reaching that decision how should the court treat the decisions of parents? I would gratefully adopt the words of Sir Thomas Bingham M.R. in *In re Z (A Minor) (Identification: Restrictions on Publication)* [1997] Fam. 1, 32–33, where he said:

> "I would for my part accept without reservation that the decision of a devoted and responsible parent should be treated with respect. It should certainly not be disregarded or lightly set aside. But the role of the court is to exercise an independent and objective judgment. If that judgment is in accord with that of the devoted and responsible parent, well and good. If it is not, then it is the duty of the court, after giving due weight to the view of the devoted and responsible parent, to give effect to its own judgment. That is what it is there for. Its judgment may of course be wrong. So may that of the parent. But once the jurisdiction of the court is invoked its clear duty is to reach and express the best judgment it can."

The issue then is what is in the best interests of the child? One factor in determining that issue to be taken into account by the court is the decision of devoted and responsible parents. It is, I would suggest, misleading to ask, once it is accepted that the parents are devoted and responsible, whether their decision is reasonable or unreasonable because parents who are responsible and devoted will almost certainly reach a decision which falls within the range of decisions which

can be classed as reasonable. If the decision falls outside the range of permissible decisions, it is unlikely that the parents are responsible and devoted parents who have sought only to decide in the best interests of their child.

In my judgment the judge misled himself by categorising the parents' decision as being "unreasonable." I can see nothing to justify the judge's conclusion that the child's mother is deluding herself that with her care the child miraculously will survive beyond that period of time forecast by the doctors, or that the parents have failed to grasp the improvements in operating technique and subsequent treatment which have taken place in the field of liver transplantation in recent years, particularly in view of Dr. P.'s evidence of the protracted and thorough discussions he has had with the mother.

If the proper stance for parents is that, whenever there is a treatment which may prolong the life of their child, then that treatment should be accepted, a decision not to accept that treatment would be unreasonable. But in my opinion that cannot be and will not be the answer in every case. Nor are such decisions to be taken solely with medical factors in mind. The presumption in favour of the sustaining of life is not irrebuttable and perhaps has less weight where the issue is whether to prolong or not to prolong life by means of organ transplantation.

The view of the parents in a liver transplant case has two aspects. First, if, as here, the parents are devoted and responsible and have the best interests of their child in mind, then their views are to be taken into account and accorded weight and respect by the court when reaching its decision. Second, the views of the parents have a clinical significance because, in the absence of parental belief that a transplant is the right procedure for the child, the prospects of a successful outcome are diminished. This factor explains the stance adopted at hospital Y. It may also explain the passage in *Fact Sheet No. 10*, published by the Children's Liver Disease Foundation and given to the mother in this case, in which this sentence appears: "If the family choose not to proceed with the transplantation once they are acquainted with the facts, this decision is respected."

I have formed the view that the judge was wrong to categorise the parents' decision as unreasonable and to disregard it in the balancing exercise he had to perform; the judge, therefore, misdirected himself, and we, in this court, should exercise the court's inherent jurisdiction.

There are formidable practical difficulties in this case which stand in the way of implementing the order which the judge in fact made. The child's father works abroad. The mother and the child and the father at present are living together. If the mother does not comply with the order, it is not certain whether the courts of the country in which they live will assist in any proceedings to oblige the mother to comply or how long such proceedings would take. The order involves the child and the mother returning to this country, although the financial ability of the family to pay for that is uncertain, particularly if it is necessary for a doctor to accompany the child during the journey. The return of the child to this country must involve both mother and child in distress which will arise from leaving the father and their home, and that must in turn increase the risk that such a journey poses for this child. On arrival in this country it is clear that the operation could not be performed at hospital Y, the hospital that the mother would choose were she disposed to seek a transplant for her child, because that hospital will not perform such an operation without the mother's willing consent. There is another possible centre at

which such an operation might be performed, hospital Z. Whereas the surgeon at that centre has indicated that he would be prepared to perform such an operation although the mother was not consenting, it is not clear whether the remainder of the medical team at that centre would be of his view or whether they would take the view set out in *Fact Sheet No 10*.

Then there is the question of treatment following the operation. Are the mother and child to stay in this country? If they are to stay for how long? If further transplant operations become necessary will the mother give or withhold her consent? What will be the position if at such time the mother and child have returned to country AB?

At present the evidence indicates that this child has a happy and secure life with his parents in country AB. It is true that that life will be a very short life which will end when the child is still a baby, but at a time before the child can become aware of the significance of his condition and its consequences. I do not consider that it is in the child's best interests to disrupt his present life by the court giving its consent to his undergoing a liver transplant operation and ordering the mother to return with him to this country with all the distress and uncertainties that that will inevitably entail for the child in the special circumstances that exist in this case.

I agree that this appeal should be allowed.

Appeal allowed.

Order of judge set aside.

Guardian ad litem refused leave to appeal.

Solicitors: Pannone & Partners; Solicitor for the local authority; Official Solicitor.

H. D.

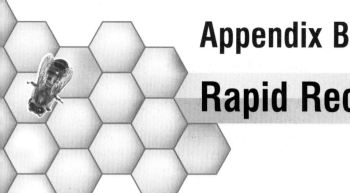

Appendix B

Rapid Recap – answers

Chapter 1

1. What are values?

1. Values are ideals, beliefs, customs and characteristics that an individual, or a particular group or society, consider valuable and worthwhile. Values are part of who you are and what makes you unique. They influence your behaviour and help you make choices and decisions. They also provide you with a frame of reference so that you can understand and evaluate new experiences and relationships.

2. How can you identify a moral issue?

2. You can identify a moral issue when a question arises about a person's rights, duties or obligations, or you need to make a judgement about the 'rightness' or 'wrongness' of a situation or a set of circumstances.

3. Give one reason why is it important to study ethics.

3. It is important to study ethics for the following reasons:
   a. The number and complexity of ethical dilemmas that you are likely to encounter in health-care settings are inevitably going to be greater than those faced by ordinary members of the public in their everyday lives.
   b. Your patients and clients may be very vulnerable.
   c. You are likely to come into contact with people from a wide variety of ethnic, cultural and religious backgrounds.

4. Give one reason why we need law.

4. We need law to:
   a. Maintain public order
   b. Facilitate co-operative action
   c. Remedy grievances

   d. Constitute and control the principal organs of power.

5. Distinguish between legislation and case law.

5. *Legislation* comprises primary legislation – i.e. Acts of Parliament – and secondary legislation – i.e. typically Statutory Instruments, usually in the form of Rules and Regulations. *Case law* is also known as common law, whereby decisions are made by judges, who create laws for later judges to follow.

Chapter 2

1. What are the founding principles of the NHS?

1. a. It should be a tax-funded service.
   b. It should provide universal health care.
   c. It should be free at the point of use to those in need.

2. Why are Primary Care Trusts (PCTs) referred to as the cornerstone of the NHS?

2. Because they not only control 75% of the NHS budget but are locally based and so are in the best position to understand the needs of the community.

3. What are the big themes that characterise New Labour's NHS reforms?

3. a. Modernisation
   b. Consumerism
   c. Privatisation
   d. Quality.

4. What does the term 'clinical governance' mean?

4. Clinical governance is the framework through which the 'quality' can be maintained throughout the NHS; in other words it is a way of guaranteeing that health-care services are the 'best that are available'.

Chapter 3

1. What does 'rationing' mean?

1. 'Rationing' means a process or mechanism for setting priorities in health care bearing in mind that resources cannot be provided to everyone who demands them.

2. What is distributive justice?

2. Distributive justice is concerned with making sure that individuals receive care and treatment that is appropriate and proper, i.e. that health-care resources are shared out 'fairly'.

3. Define the QALY approach to the allocation of resources.

3. The QALY (quality adjusted life years) approach aims to calculate the most efficient use of resources that will improve the quality of people's lives over the longest period of time.

4. What legal options can a patient use if they are denied treatment?

3. If a patient is denied treatment, s/he can use the following legal options:
   a. Judicial review
   b. Breach of statutory duty/negligence.

5. What obligations are imposed on the Secretary of State under the National Health Service Act 1977?

5. Under the Act, the Secretary of State is obliged to provide:
   a. A comprehensive health service (in England and Wales) designed to secure improvement in the physical and mental health of people and the prevention, diagnosis and treatment of illness
   b. Hospital and community services as well as primary health care.

Chapter 4

1. What is 'professional law'?

1. The regulation of professional practice by regulatory bodies.

2. What are the main functions of codes of professional conduct?

2. To:
   a. Set, maintain and improve ethical standards
   b. Regulate ethical professional conduct

c. Provide information
d. Encourage a common identity.

3. What do the NMC and HPC do?

3. They are statutory bodies for professionals qualified in the health-care professions. The NMC:
   a. Maintains a register listing all nurses, midwives and health visitors
   b. Sets standards and guidelines for education, practice and conduct
   c. Provides advice on professional standards
   d. Assures quality education
   e. Sets standards and guidelines for local supervising authorities for midwives
   f. Considers allegations of misconduct or unfitness to practise due to ill health.

The HPC:
   a. Maintains and publishes a public register of properly qualified members of the profession
   b. Approves and upholds high standards of education and training and continued good practice
   c. Investigates complaints and takes appropriate action
   d. Works in partnership with the public and a range of other groups
   e. Promotes awareness and understanding of the aims of the Council.

4. How is a health professional's 'fitness to practise' impaired?

4. By misconduct, lack of competence, ill health or criminal convictions or cautions.

5. What is the Council for the Regulation of Health Care Professionals?

5. It is an independent body that oversees the work of existing regulating health-care professional bodies.

Chapter 5

1. What are the functions of negligence law?

1. a. Compensation
   b. Deterrence
   c. Retribution
   d. Investigation.

2. Which ethical principles form the moral foundations of your code of professional conduct?

2. Beneficence, i.e. the duty to care, and non-maleficence, i.e. the duty not to harm others.

3. What is the difference between responsibility and accountability

3. Accountability means that you must justify your actions (i.e. explain why you behaved as you did) whereas responsibility either describes your role or indicates that you have caused something to happen.

4. What are the elements of a negligence claim?

4. a. A duty of care that is owed
   b. The defendant has breached that duty
   c. Damage.

5. What is the Bolam test?

5. The general legal principle that practitioners who have acted in the same way as other reasonably competent members of their profession will not normally be found to have been negligent.

Chapter 6

1. What does respect for autonomy mean?

1. To acknowledge a person's right to hold views, make choices and take actions based on personal values and beliefs.

2. Why is autonomy important?

2. Because it reflects the modern moral and political philosophy of:
   a. Freedom for the individual
   b. Human rights
   c. An equal relationship between health professionals and patients.

3. What are the essential elements of legal consent?

3. For consent to be legally valid you must make sure that:
   a. It is voluntary
   b. Enough information has been given and
   c. The patient is competent.

4. What is the legal consequence of not giving patient adequate information?

4. That you could face a negligence claim.

5. How are decisions made for patients who are incompetent?

5. Adult patients who are incompetent because they are unconscious can be treated under the doctrine of necessity, i.e. treatment can be carried out that is necessary to save the patient's life and health.

Other adult patients who are incompetent can be treated without their consent as long as the treatment is in their best interests.

Chapter 7

1. What is confidentiality?

1. The principle of keeping secure and secret from others information by or about an individual that you have come by in the course of a professional relationship.

2. Why is confidentiality important?

2. Because of:
   a. The future consequences if confidentiality is not maintained
   b. Respect for patient autonomy.

3. What is the purpose of the 2003 NHS confidentiality code of practice?

3. a. To introduce the concept of confidentiality
   b. To describe what a confidential service looks like
   c. To provide a description of the main legal requirements
   d. To recommend a generic decision support tool for sharing/disclosing information
   e. To list examples of particular information-sharing experiences.

4. Is confidentiality an absolute principle?

4. No, confidentiality is not an absolute principle, i.e. it can be broken.

5. What is meant by the 'public interest'?

5. The interests of an individual or groups of individuals or of society as a whole.

Chapter 8

1. Distinguish between therapeutic and non-therapeutic research.

1. Therapeutic research aims to benefit the patients whereas non-therapeutic research aims to gain scientific knowledge.

2. What are the key ethical principles underpinning research?

2. a. Respect for autonomy
   b. Justice
   c. Beneficence and non-maleficence
   d. Scientific validity.

3. **What are the main aims of the NHS Research Governance Framework 2004?**

3. To improve research quality and to safeguard the public.

4. **What is the main purpose of an REC?**

4. To form an independent review to vet the ethical aspects of research.

5. **How does the law regulate research?**

5. By relying on the law of consent.

Chapter 9

1. **What is the role of the HFEA?**

1. To safeguard, protect and reassure patients, professionals and the public about licensed fertility treatments and human embryo research.

2. **The regulation of assisted conception has two main purposes: what are they?**

2. a. To ensure that the techniques are safe
   b. To ensure that their use is ethical.

3. **What is the main aim of prenatal genetic testing?**

3. To investigate individual pregnancies where the foetus because of a specified reason is judged to be at an increased risk of a genetic condition.

4. **What does the phrase 'maternal immunity' mean?**

4. That a mother cannot be sued by her children for injuries sustained during pregnancy.

5. **Can a competent pregnant woman be forced to have a caesarean?**

5. No, she cannot be legally forced to have a caesarean. This was emphatically confirmed in the case of *Re M.B.* (1997), when the judge said that a competent pregnant woman has the absolute legal right to refuse all treatment (including a caesarean) whatever the consequences to her or the foetus.

Chapter 10

1. **Is the foetus a legal person?**

1. No. This was established in the case of *Re F.* (1988), which confirmed that it is only after birth,

i.e. once a baby is born alive, that it acquires independent legal status separate from that of its mother.

2. **What is meant by the phrase: 'the foetus has a right to life'?**

2. That a foetus has the same moral claims as a person and thus the right not to be deliberately killed.

3. **When is an abortion legal?**

3. When it is performed by a registered medical practitioner after two registered medical practitioners have decided 'in good faith' the one or more grounds specified in the Abortion Act 1967 apply.

4. **What is a 'wrongful birth' claim?**

4. A claim for damages for the following reasons:
   a. Failure to detect foetal abnormality
   b. Giving a pregnant woman incorrect information about the results of a prenatal test
   c. Assisted conception (if a disabled child is born as a result of inadequate screening of donor gametes).

Chapter 11

1. **How can you justify the compulsory detention and treatment of patients with mental disorders?**

1. By your moral obligation to protect the public and to protect the mentally ill from themselves.

2. **What does 'sectioning' mean?**

2. The compulsory detainment of patients.

3. **What does the phrase 'informal admission' mean?**

3. Admission of a patient into psychiatric care without the use of compulsory powers.

4. **Can patients be force-fed?**

4. Yes – patients can be force-fed under both the Mental Health Act 1983 and the common law.

5. **When is treatment of patients with learning disabilities lawful?**

1. Such treatment is lawful providing it complies with the 'best interests' test.

Chapter 12

1. What is the Gillick test?

1. The Gillick test assesses whether under 16-year-olds can independently consent to treatment or to take part in research.

2. Why is it important to know who has parental responsibility?

2. Because it is this person who will legally be able to give consent.

3. When can parents give consent to research on their children?

3. When they are not Gillick-competent.

4. What does 'significant harm' mean?

4. Ill-treatment or the impairment of health or development that is considerable or important.

Chapter 13

1. What does the word 'ageism' mean?

1. The stereotyping of and discrimination against older people.

2. What is the NSF for older people?

2. A government document that aims to stop age discrimination in health and social care settings by setting new national standards of care for all older people.

3. What is the fair innings argument?

3. That older people have had their fair share of health care and so should give up their place in the queue (for an operation or medical procedure) to younger patients.

4. What is elder abuse?

4. The mistreatment of an older person.

5. Is it lawful to restrain a 'wandering' incompetent older person?

5. Yes, provided that it is temporary and that it is the only way to prevent the patient injuring him/herself or someone else.

Chapter 14

1. What is the sanctity of life doctrine?

1. The belief that human life is sacred and that taking it is wrong, therefore euthanasia is wrong.

2. What is the principle of double effect?

2. The principle that something that we do in order to produce a good effect may also simultaneously have a harmful effect and that, even although the harmful effect can be foreseen, if it is not intended the action that it produces is not wrong.

3. What is a DNR order?

3. A direction that in the event of a cardiac arrest neither basic nor advanced life support measures should be started.

4. What is an advance directive?

4. A statement made by an adult, at a time when they are competent, about how they want to be treated in the future should they become ill and no longer able to make decisions or communicate their wishes.

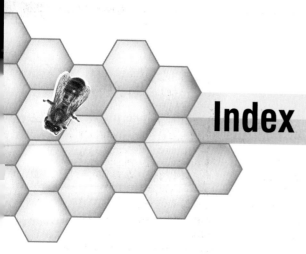

Index